D0405683

THE Mediterranean HEART DIET

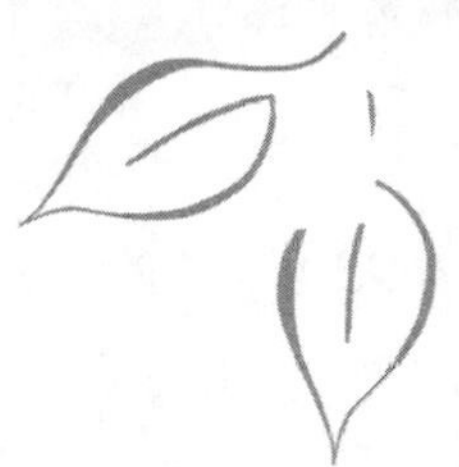

Why It Works, with Recipes to Get You Started

HELEN V. FISHER
WITH CYNTHIA THOMSON, PH.D., R.D.,
AND KAJA LEWINN

PERSEUS PUBLISHING
Cambridge, Massachusetts

Cataloging-in-Publication data for this book is available from the Library of Congress.
ISBN 1-55561-281-4

Perseus Publishing is a member of the Perseus Books Group.
Find us on the World Wide Web at http://www.perseuspublishing.com

Perseus Publishing books are available at special discounts for bulk purchases in the United States by corporations, institutions and other organizations. For more information, please contact the Special Markets Department at the Perseus Books Group, 11 Cambridge Center, Cambridge, MA 02142, or call (617) 252-5298.

Text design by Tonya Hahn
Set in 11-point Fairfield Light by Perseus Publishing Services

First printing, June 2001
2 3 4 5 6 7 8 9 10—04 03 02 01

Contents

Part 1: The Mediterranean Heart Diet: A Healthful Approach to Eating

by Cynthia Thomson, Ph.D., R.D., and Kaja LeWinn

Part 2: Easy-to-Prepare Recipes for the Mediterranean Diet

The Mediterranean Heart Diet: A Healthful Approach to Eating

Cynthia Thomson, R.D., Ph.D., and Kaja LeWinn

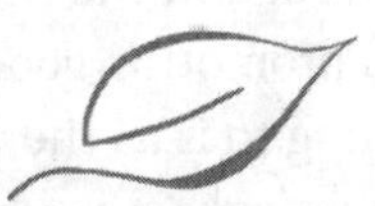

What Is the Mediterranean Heart Diet?

What we know as the Mediterranean diet focuses on foods traditionally consumed by people living around the sparkling Mediterranean Sea, whose daily fare traditionally includes plenty of fresh fruits and colorful vegetables, hearty whole grains and legumes, olive oil, yogurt, cheese, a little fish, at least six 8-ounce glasses of water, often flavored with citrus peel, and a touch of wine. Foods that conform to a Mediterranean-style diet are full of flavor, easy to prepare, and—because they emphasize unprocessed foods and include only small amounts of meat as a seasoning rather than as the main course—inexpensive. But these inviting attributes aren't the only reasons that this cuisine has caught the world's attention.

Medical studies beginning more than fifty years ago observed that the people living in the Mediterranean area, particularly in Greece, were much less likely than those in industrialized societies to develop heart disease or suffer strokes. They were also less likely to develop certain cancers, become overweight, or develop diabetes. Scientists were curious—why was this so? Diet was soon identified as a major reason for the good health and long lives that the Mediterranean peoples enjoyed, and the Mediterranean diet became associated in particular with promoting good heart health. We emphasize this fact by referring to it as the "Mediterranean Heart Diet" in this book. Lots of physical activity—walking to visit neighbors, tending small farms, bicycling to town—was another important component of the overall lifestyle that conferred good health.

Today health experts have amassed a powerful array of evidence in favor of following a Mediterranean-style diet and lifestyle, and they continue to find new health benefits in the foods the diet emphasizes. We will discuss these benefits in detail later in this chapter and will tell you everything you need to know to start enjoying more healthful and flavorful meals right away. But first, let's take a look at the dietary features that make this eating plan special, and at the medical-research findings that support it.

Foods of the Mediterranean

The Mediterranean region is noted for simple yet delicious meals centered around seasonal vegetables and fruits, hearty breads, pasta, rice, and legumes, supplemented with olive oil, small amounts of nuts, cheese, and yogurt, and occasionally meat. Each area—from Greece and Italy to northern Africa and the coasts of France and Spain—shares these traits, even though each places a slightly different emphasis on certain ingredients, such as pasta or rice or a certain type of legume. This book provides recipes that reflect the Mediterranean to start you on your way to delicious, healthful eating.

Grains, Pasta, and Rice

The Mediterranean diet emphasizes complex carbohydrates—the ones from whole grains and starches, not sugar. Complex carbohydrates in the Mediterranean diet are found in whole-grain hearty breads made without eggs or fat, pasta, rice, bulgur (cracked whole wheat), polenta made from coarse cornmeal, couscous (a form of pasta eaten in North Africa) and potatoes. These foods provide most of the energy (calories) in the diet. In addition, they contribute good amounts of fiber, protein, B vitamins, and minerals. The number of daily servings required from this food group depends on the amount of energy an individual needs to maintain his or her ideal body weight, but follow this rule of thumb: Your plate should be mostly filled with foods from this group. A general guide is probably 2 to 3 cups of pasta or rice with three or more servings of whole-grain breads daily. Couscous Fruit Salad (page 88) is an example of a dish with good amounts of fiber and complex carbohydrates.

> Your plate should be mostly filled with foods from this group.

Vegetables, Fruits, Legumes, and Nuts

The food group of next importance contains vegetables, fruits, legumes, and nuts. Vegetables are an essential part of the diet in the Mediterranean; they compose the largest part of the diet after complex carbohydrates. The selection is staggering, ranging from artichokes to eggplant, kale to rapini (broccoli rabe), tomatoes to zucchini—no need to settle for the starchy corn and peas that have been vegetable staples for too many of us!

The freshest vegetables come from home gardens; the next best from farmer's markets or vegetable stands in cities. The key to

The key to selecting both vegetables and fruits is to follow the example of the Mediterranean peoples: Choose what is fresh, seasonal, and in the best condition.

selecting vegetables and fruits is to follow the example of the Mediterranean peoples: Choose what is fresh, seasonal, and in the best condition. (Ask your grocer for advice at first if you need to.) Vegetables are eaten both raw and cooked and appear throughout the menu—in soups, salads, main dishes, side dishes, and appetizers. Salads in the Mediterranean are diverse and bursting with flavor from many kinds of salad greens and other vegetables. Now is the time to leave behind those flavorless salads made from limp iceberg lettuce and pale tomatoes!

Vegetables provide fiber; several vitamins, including folate (folic acid), vitamin C, and vitamin A; minerals such as calcium and iron; and some protein in the diet, while contributing few calories. Include dark leafy and bright orange and yellow vegetables such as kale, broccoli, rapini, cabbage, squash, carrots, and tomatoes in your selection; consume five or six servings of vegetables per day. Remember, a serving size for most vegetables is just half a cup. If you feel that eating six different vegetables a day is overwhelming, just select two or three to eat and boost the portion size. For example, that Mediterranean salad on the menu at your local restaurant in most cases is at least as large as two—and many times, three—servings. Choose a salad such as Marinated Dates and Figs with Spinach and Fennel (page 89) for a delicious way to get lots of fiber and wonderful flavor. Recipes for members of the cabbage family (the cruciferous vegetables) are included in the Vegetables chapter. Try Cauliflower in Mustard Sauce (page 188) or Brussels Sprouts with Currants and Walnuts (page 189).

Fruits are eaten raw as snacks or for dessert with perhaps a small slice of cheese. They are sometimes eaten dried or poached in a little wine and sugar for a dessert. (Desserts that are more elaborate, such as cakes and cookies, are reserved for special occasions.) Fruits provide fiber, vitamin C, and other antioxidants, such as beta-carotene, in the diet—important nutrients in preventing heart disease. Choose two to three servings of fruit per day, mostly in the form of whole fruit with its juice. Choose some orange-colored fruits, such as cantaloupe, mangoes, and oranges, because they are higher in health-promoting carotenoids, of which beta-carotene is the most familiar example. Occasionally want more than just a piece of fruit at the end of a meal? Try Fruit Medley with Honey-Yogurt Sauce (page 216) for a tasty change of pace.

Legumes such as lentils, white beans, fava beans, and garbanzo beans (chickpeas) are used in soups, salads, and main dishes. They provide much of the protein in the diet and contribute good amounts of fiber—especially the soluble fiber that helps prevent heart disease—minerals, B vitamins, and energy. Eat 1 cup of cooked legumes daily. Lentils with Vegetables (page 135) is a delicious way to prepare lentils, or try Beans, Rice, and Vegetables (page 121). Both dishes can be served as a main course. In Italy, pasta and beans make a classic combination as a main course.

Nuts provide fiber, protein, and other nutrients, such as vitamin E and calcium. Nuts are not often considered part of a healthful diet because they are high in fat, but the fat that they contribute is "good" fat that contains many of the essential fatty acids needed for good health. Include small amounts of nuts when planning your menus. Many recipes throughout this book include a sprinkling of nuts to add flavor and crunch, along with good fats and vitamin E, to your meals.

> Vegetables are an essential part of the diet in the Mediterranean; they compose the largest part of the diet after carbohydrates.

Olive Oil

One important element that distinguishes the cuisine of the Mediterranean from others is the generous use of olive oil in both cooking and at the table. It almost completely replaces the saturated fats such as butter, margarine, and vegetable shortening used in other parts of the world. (Butter is used in small amounts in some special-occasion desserts.) Olive oil is used for cooking, for dressing salads, and at the table on bread and is sometimes drizzled over finished dishes to add flavor. Olive oil is mostly monounsaturated fat

> Olive oil is mostly monounsaturated fat, which is known to help prevent heart disease.

(see the "Types of Fat and Sources" box on page 19), which is known to help prevent heart disease. The amount of olive oil that you use will depend on your daily energy (calorie) requirements, but a good guideline is to *replace* all the fats that you use in cooking, on salads, and at the table with olive oil—probably a minimum of 2 tablespoons per day. An easy way to get more olive oil in your diet is to use it in a salad dressing, such as Balsamic Herb Dressing (page 103).

Dairy Products

Milk is not consumed as a beverage in the Mediterranean, but dairy products aren't neglected in the diet. Small amounts of mostly robust cheeses add zest to many dishes and are also eaten in small amounts with fruit. These are probably the main sources of saturated fat in the diet, and they are always eaten in moderation. In many parts of the Mediterranean, at least 1 cup of yogurt is eaten daily and is a major source of calcium in the diet. In our country, yogurt can be used for breakfast and spooned over fruits and vegetables at other meals. Make your own Yogurt Cream Cheese (page 62), or try yogurt in Cucumber-Yogurt Dressing (page 109).

Fish and Poultry

Fish and poultry are consumed more frequently than red meat, but still in limited amounts compared to practices in North America. Fish is an important source of omega-3 fatty acids, which are important in preventing heart disease. Fish is also a desirable source of low-fat protein.

> Fish is an important source of omega-3 fatty acids, which are important in preventing heart disease.

The Mediterranean peoples have traditionally raised poultry, which, unlike raising cattle, requires little in the way of space or forage. Like beef, meat from poultry provides flavor and lean protein to the diet. Eat fish and poultry at two to four meals per week as a "main course" (3-ounce servings), or more frequently if you use it in smaller amounts. Try Baked Cod and Tomatoes over Brown Rice (page 142) or Sweet and Spicy Chicken with Peaches (page 166).

Eggs, Sweets, and Red Meats

The foods eaten least frequently in the Mediterranean diet are eggs, sweets, and red meats. Eggs are used in some breads and special desserts but do not have a regular place on the breakfast table. As mentioned, sweets are reserved for special occasions.

Traditionally, lamb and pork are the most popular meats on the menu, with beef eaten only occasionally. Like desserts, large amounts of meat, such as roasts, are associated with special occasions. As a rule, meats are eaten as a condiment mixed with vegetables or pasta—not as the main ingredient—in much the same way that we use onions or garlic for flavor. Meats contain useful amounts of fat, protein, minerals, and vitamins. It's best to eat lamb, pork, and beef only rarely as a main dish (3-ounce servings). Use them more frequently than this only to season a dish (less than 1 ounce per person).

As a rule, meats are eaten as a condiment mixed with vegetables or pasta.

For a special meal, try vegetable-packed Veal Stew (page 178). Perhaps you could do as those in the Mediterranean do for special occasions, combining nuts and olive oil in delicious, easy-to-make Orange-Walnut Semolina Cake (page 223). This heavenly cake will add just the right touch of the Mediterranean to an important meal.

Wine

The moderate consumption of wine, which is optional in the Mediterranean diet but very much part of the cuisine of the

Mediterranean, is a practice that has been endorsed by leading cardiologists. Both the antioxidants (see Antioxidants, page 22) and the alcohol in wine seem to help prevent heart disease. It is important to note that wine is consumed with food in the presence of family and friends, a feature of the Mediterranean lifestyle that helps control overconsumption. Limit daily wine intake to 1 glass for women and less than 3 for men.

It is not recommended that you begin drinking wine for this benefit if you do not drink alcohol already. If you are pregnant or nursing, you should not drink wine at all. The health risks in these cases outweigh the potential health benefit. A diet high in vegetables and fruit, particularly those rich in folate, helps control the detrimental health effects of alcohol.

In summary, the diet of the Mediterranean region is traditionally high in whole-grain breads, pasta, rice, and other grains and includes a wide array of vegetables, legumes, and fruits, along with olive oil, a little fish and poultry, and the wines of the region. Foods are fresh, minimally processed, and cooked in ways that add flavor and preserve wholesomeness. This is the diet that attracted the interest of scientists and formed the basis of what is now known as the Mediterranean diet.

The Science Behind the Mediterranean Heart Diet

In the 1950s, the role of diet in human health was a mystery. Most researchers accepted that there was a connection between diet and disease, but the nature of this connection was largely unstudied in human populations. In 1958, a young man named Ancel Keyes, from the University of Minnesota, and a team of international researchers set out to solve the mystery.

Keyes theorized that saturated fat intake could increase the risk of heart disease. He developed this hypothesis after observing that wartime shortages of meat and dairy products in Europe were associated with dramatically *decreased* rates of heart disease. He also noticed, while on a tour of Africa and Europe, that affluent people who ate a lot of rich (fatty) meat and dairy products had higher blood cholesterol levels and suffered a greater risk of heart disease than poorer people who could afford only limited amounts of these foods.

The Seven Countries Study

To test his hypothesis, Keyes and his colleagues studied a group of more than 12,000 men between the ages of 40 and 59 from seven countries: Yugoslavia, Greece, Italy, Japan, Finland, the Netherlands, and the United States. The men were enrolled between 1958 and 1964 in sixteen study groups, or cohorts. The researchers began by examining the dietary habits, physical activity, blood pressure, and serum cholesterol of this population and went on to record incidences of and deaths due to coronary heart disease (CHD) after five, ten, fifteen, and twenty years. The researchers hypothesized that the frequency of heart attacks and strokes in a given population would vary in relation to each group's physical characteristics and lifestyle patterns—and more specifically, their eating patterns.

Wartime shortages of meat and dairy products in Europe were associated with dramatically *decreased* rates of heart disease.

Ten years after the study began, researchers found that the Greek population had the lowest mortality rate from *all* causes. In addition, they found a stark difference in mortality rates due to heart disease. Finnish men had the highest incidence of heart disease, at 28 percent of the total population. Notably, this group consumed 38 percent of their calories from fat and also consumed the most saturated fat (mostly in the form of butter and cheese), at 24 percent of their total calorie intake—double what today's average American consumes! Japanese men consumed the least amount of fat (9 percent of calories) and saturated fat (3 percent of calories), and only 5 percent of this cohort developed heart disease. Clearly, the Japanese fared far better than the Finns; however, one group was even less subject to developing heart disease.

Over the same ten-year period, only 2 percent of the Greek men developed heart disease, and not one man died. The curious thing about this result was that the Greek men ate just as much total fat as the Finns; however, the fat was of a different type. Only about 8 percent of their fat intake was saturated, compared with a

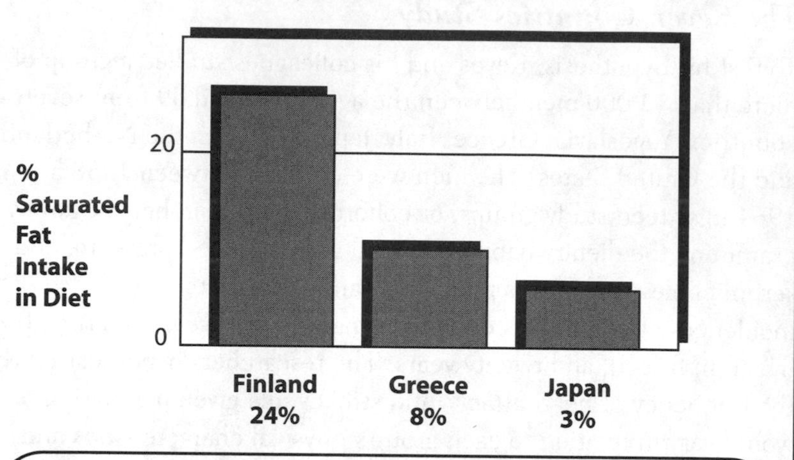

Saturated fat intake (percentage of total calories) of men in Greece, Finland, and Japan participating in the Seven Countries Study.

Changes Since the 1950s

The Mediterranean diet that has been associated with reduced heart disease and cancer risk is the one that typically existed in the Mediterranean about fifty years ago. In recent years, the dietary practices of this region have changed dramatically as a result of economic and political stability. People of this region are consuming more meat and processed foods, which were not part of the health-promoting diet of the 1950s. For this reason, the recipes in this book refer to what is known as the *traditional* Mediterranean diet, absent the recent changes in the dietary practices of this region.

whopping 24 percent among the Finns. The Japanese diet was lower still in fat; however, this group suffered a higher incidence of heart disease than did the Greeks.

How could the Greek men eat so much fat without developing heart disease? First, the researchers examined the men's blood

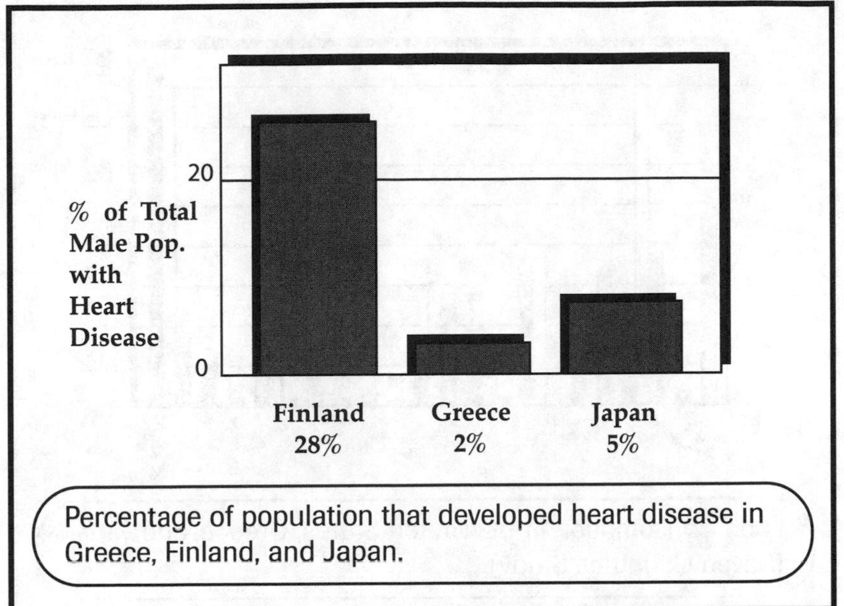

Percentage of population that developed heart disease in Greece, Finland, and Japan.

(serum) cholesterol levels. Despite their high intake of fat, Greek men had the lowest serum cholesterol levels of all seven cohorts. Evidence at that time suggested the low serum cholesterol levels were largely determined by the low intake of saturated fat and cholesterol. Further research on the associations between heart disease, saturated fat, and cholesterol has supported these findings. Reducing consumption of saturated fat and cholesterol does reduce heart-disease risk (see the figures above).

The Seven Countries Study showed that people following a traditional Mediterranean diet consume very low amounts of saturated fats, including the trans form (see the "Trans Fats" box, page 21), and high amounts of monounsaturated fat, primarily in the form of olive oil. In fact, when Ancel Keyes and his colleagues began their study in the late 1950s, 50 to 60 percent of calories consumed by the Greeks came from olive oil and whole-grain bread *alone*. The rest came primarily from fruits, vegetables, and legumes. Meat and poultry were consumed only a few times a month, and cheese and milk in small portions, yielding low levels of saturated fat and cholesterol and high levels of monounsaturated fat in the diet. This was in stark contrast to the U.S. diet at the time, which consisted of large amounts of meat and poultry and fewer fruits and vegetables—a diet much higher in saturated fat and cholesterol, with no

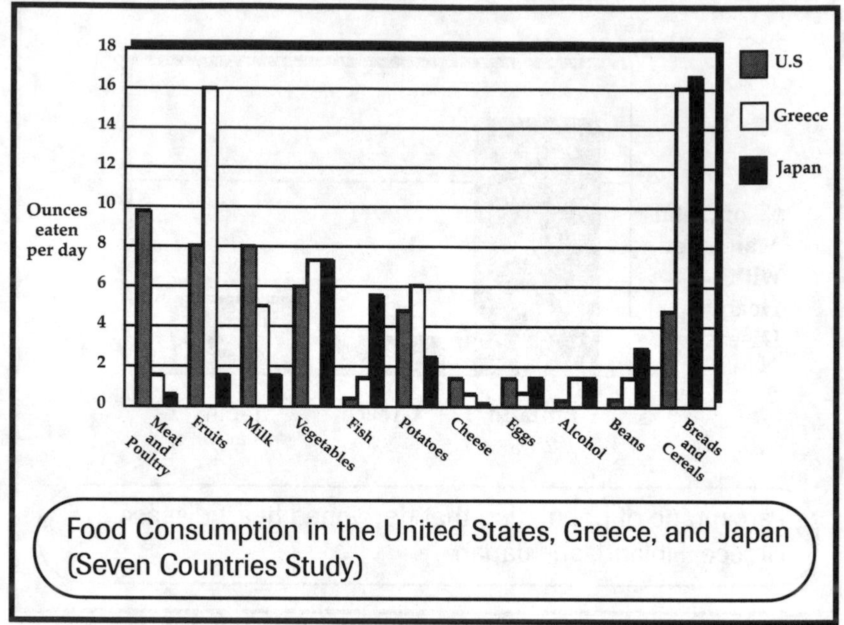

Food Consumption in the United States, Greece, and Japan (Seven Countries Study)

significant source of monounsaturated fat. The table above shows the relative consumption of certain foods in Greece, the United States, and Japan at the time Ancel Keyes conducted his research.

Another important component of the association between the Mediterranean diet and protection against heart disease is the high intake of plant foods. As the graph indicates, at the time of the Seven Countries Study, the people of Greece ate twice the amount of fruit, more vegetables, and almost three times the amount of bread and cereals as people living in the United States did.

Origins of This Healthful Cuisine

The healthful Mediterranean lifestyle, including its cuisine, probably developed out of necessity rather than choice. Unlike the United States, the Mediterranean region suffered economically following World War II which affected both the diet and physical activity of its inhabitants. While the United States could afford to consume more meat and high-fat dairy products than ever before, the people of the Mediterranean continued to consume a primarily plant-based diet, with an emphasis on local ingredients such as wheat, wine, and olive oil. The United States was able to industrialize at a rapid pace, but the people of the Mediterranean continued to till the soil without the benefit of much machinery to help them. Foods came straight from the farm; processed foods were scarce. Breads, grains, potatoes, fruits, and vegetables made up the bulk of every meal. Beans and nuts were used both for flavor and texture.

Typically, people in the Mediterranean consumed modest portions of cheese and yogurt several times a week and meat and poultry rarely. They used herbs and olive oil to transform these simple ingredients into delectable dishes that are now known around the world for their unique, lively flavors.

Why the Diet Promotes Good Health

Living close to the land, concentrating on fresh, unprocessed foods that were largely plant-based, the people of the Mediterranean created a diet high in complex carbohydrates, fiber, antioxidants, vitamins, and minerals—dietary ingredients that science has shown confer many health benefits. After World War II, and for years

Crete and the Mediterranean Lifestyle

A narrow island 152 miles long, Crete is the largest island of modern Greece, and its inhabitants provide a good example of the traditional Mediterranean lifestyle. Agriculture is the primary economic resource, although only about one-third of Crete's land can be cultivated. Farmers traditionally own small plots, on which they plant and harvest a variety of crops without the help of machinery.

The livelihood of the people of Crete is bound to the land and its products, notably olive oil. Local farmers provide the islanders with a variety of fruits, vegetables, nuts, grains, herbs, yogurt, and cheese. These simple ingredients are brought home daily and turned into a gloriously good meal. The table is typically covered with a variety of foods: fava bean soup, tomato salad, potatoes, and bread. There is a glass of wine for each adult. Food is prepared lovingly, with minimal processing, and meals are enjoyed in a leisurely way.

> The people of Greece ate twice the amount of fruit, more vegetables, and almost three times the amount of bread and cereals as did people living in the United States.

afterward, Mediterranean peoples ate limited amounts of animal products, keeping their consumption of saturated fat low. While total fat intake in the traditional diet was somewhat high (researchers observed it to be as high as 40 percent of daily calories consumed), *the type of oil consumed is significant*. Olive oil, low in saturated fat, high in monounsaturated fat, made up the bulk of total fat intake. This specific dietary combination—high in plant-based foods, low in animal products, with olive oil contributing most of the fat consumed—has proved to have the greatest protective effect against heart disease.

Physical activity is another important aspect of the Mediterranean lifestyle and is directly related to the decreased risk of heart disease and cancer in this region. Traditionally, the Mediterranean people have incorporated physical activity into their daily lives. Not all families owned a car, and people frequently walked or cycled to their destinations. They usually tended their small farms by hand, planting and harvesting a variety of crops. Physical activity *and* a good diet go hand in hand in any truly healthful lifestyle.

Healthful Benefits of the Diet

The Mediterranean Diet and Heart Disease

Heart disease is the number-one cause of death in the United States, killing more than 500,000 Americans a year. Chronic diseases (such as heart disease, cancer, diabetes, and obesity) plague Western society, although our risk of developing most of these diseases could be drastically reduced simply by changing what we eat. Thanks to the landmark Seven Countries Study, researchers learned much about the relationship between diet and heart disease. The study revealed that the Greeks had the lowest incidence of heart disease, compared to inhabitants of the six other countries in the study. Studies that have followed this one have shown that people in the Mediterranean also suffer less from high blood pressure, cancer, and obesity, diseases that continue to be a major health burden in the United States. Yet far from simply "getting by" on a bland or meager diet, the people of the Mediterranean have traditionally enjoyed a fully satisfying and flavorful one—a diet, in fact, that everyone can enjoy eating.

After linking health to eating habits, researchers went on to closely examine each component of the Mediterranean diet in an effort to find a solution to the growing problem of chronic disease in the United States. They focused on the fact that unlike other Western diets, the Mediterranean diet was primarily plant-based; rich in fruits, vegetables, and whole grains; and high in antioxidants and other nutrients. They found that the diet was virtually free of saturated fat, because the people consumed very little red meat or dairy products and used olive oil (a monounsaturated fat) as their primary fat source. They also found that many people in the Mediterranean drank one or two glasses of wine almost every day. Each of these intriguing findings prompted investigations of their own.

Fat in the Mediterranean Diet

Olive Oil and Total Fat Intake. As we have noted, a major dietary ingredient that distinguishes the cuisine of the Mediterranean is olive oil, which is used liberally in cooking and at the table. It almost completely replaces the saturated fats such as butter, margarine, and vegetable shortening used in other parts of the world. Olive oil is used for cooking, dressing salads, and at the table on bread, and is sometimes drizzled over finished dishes to add flavor. Olive oil is mostly monounsaturated fat, the kind that increases the amount of HDL, the "good" cholesterol circulating in the bloodstream, and decreases triglyceride levels in the blood, reducing the risk of heart disease. (For a discussion of the role these substances play in heart health, see the "Cholesterol and Triglycerides" box, page 16.)

> Physical activity is a key factor in the reduction of chronic disease and is a vital part of the Mediterranean lifestyle.

Olive oil is used almost exclusively as fat in the

Cholesterol and Triglycerides

Cholesterol is an essential element in the human body. Without it, we would not survive. It is used in the synthesis of hormones (such as estrogen, testosterone, and progesterone) and is an important structural element in cell membranes. Cholesterol circulates in the bloodstream in large complexes called lipoproteins.

There are five types of lipoproteins, two of which are implicated in the development or prevention of heart disease: high-density lipoproteins (HDL) and low-density lipoproteins (LDL). LDL is the major carrier of cholesterol in the bloodstream and is harmless if levels are maintained within a certain range. If LDL levels are high, however, these molecules become targets for free radicals. Free radicals are molecules with one unpaired, or "free," electron that can bind to other molecules and destabilize them in a process called oxidation. That is where problems can begin.

When free radicals bind to the LDL molecule, they are transformed into something the body doesn't recognize. The body reacts by attacking the oxidized LDL as it would an infection, sending in white cells to overwhelm the "intruder." These groups of white cells clump together and form plaque, which can block the flow of blood through an artery over time. (This process is called atherosclerosis, also known as hardening of the arteries.) This plaque decreases the flow of blood-borne oxygen to the heart or brain, contributing to the development of coronary artery disease and increasing the risk of stroke. A heart attack occurs when plaque fully blocks a coronary artery. One type of stroke occurs when plaque blocks an artery that supplies blood to the brain, causing brain damage to the area that is not receiving oxygen. Risk of both stroke and heart disease are lowered when plaque formation is reduced.

HDL has quite a different function in the body. It binds to excess cholesterol in the cells and helps to transport it to the liver. Because HDL removes excess cholesterol from the bloodstream, thus reducing the risk of heart attack and stroke, it is known as the "good" cholesterol. (In contrast, LDL is sometimes referred to as "bad," or "lousy," cholesterol.) Recent research indicates that raising HDL levels may be just as important as lowering LDL levels in preventing heart disease.

Triglycerides are another form of fat. They are carried in the blood by the very low density lipoproteins (VLDLs). Like cholesterol, they can be deposited on arterial walls and cause blockages. Elevated levels of triglycerides in the blood can also increase the possibility of blood clots and therefore the risk of heart disease. Eating a lot of sugary foods, other refined carbohydrates, and fat, and indulging in excess alcohol consumption, can elevate triglyceride levels quickly. Circulating blood triglyceride levels rise following a high-fat meal, for example.

Suggested Cholesterol and Triglyceride Levels

	Low-Risk Group	High-Risk Group (family history of heart disease, smoking, high blood pressure)
Total cholesterol	200mg/dl or below	200mg/dl or below
LDL	160mg/dl or below	130mg/dl or below
HDL	Women: 50mg/dl; Men: 45mg/dl	60mg/dl may be high enough to cancel out a risk factor
Triglycerides	150mg/dl	100mg/dl

mg/dl = milligram per deciliter

Mediterranean diet, and the percentage of calories from fat in the diet often exceeds the 30 percent recommended in North American eating plans. This is less a cause for concern than it first appears, because saturated-fat consumption is assumed as part of a typical North American diet. Saturated fats should be limited in the diet because they form LDL cholesterol, which increases the risk for heart disease. Monounsaturated fats, like olive oil, do not have this effect.

Note: We do not recommend consuming 40 percent of calories from fat, even if it is unsaturated. Fat is still extremely high in calories and Americans who are not physically active easily gain weight if they increase their total fat intake. For this reason, the recipes in this book have been designed to include only 30 percent fat, mostly from monounsaturated sources such as olive oil, nuts, and seeds.

As we noted previously, diets high in monounsaturated fat have been shown to increase the level of HDL ("good" cholesterol) and decrease triglyceride levels in the bloodstream, thereby reducing heart-disease risk. A diet high in olive oil has other benefits, too.

- Olive oil is lower in linolenic acid (omega-6) than other vegetable oils. Linolenic acid may compete with omega-3 fatty acids, which reduce the tendency of blood to clot.
- Some animal studies have found that diets high in polyunsaturated fat promote tumor development. Substituting olive oil or other sources of monounsaturated fat for polyunsaturated fat in the diet may therefore be better for health.
- Olive oil is high in vitamin E, the antioxidant most associated with heart-disease prevention.

Unlike monounsaturated fat, saturated fat has been associated with increased breast, colon, and prostate cancer risk. Recent evidence indicates that colon cancer may be related to meat consumption. In addition, when meat is cooked at high temperatures, as it is frequently (for example, by frying or grilling), a group of chemicals (heterocyclic amines) are produced. These chemicals have the potential to create abnormal cells and increase cancer risk.

However, fat is not "all bad"; it plays an important role in good health, because cells require fat to function normally. A small amount of fat in the diet helps you to feel full and satisfied after eating a meal. Fat is also important for the absorption of the fat-soluble vitamins A, D, E, and K and many of the protective phytochemicals, including carotenoids (phytochemicals are discussed in detail on pages 32–34).

The Relationship Between Fat Consumption and Heart Disease. Harvard University medical researchers, in another significant long-term study known as the Nurses Health Study (NHS), estimated that by replacing 5 percent of total daily calories from saturated fat with unsaturated fat, a woman's risk for heart disease could be reduced by 42 percent. Two easy ways to do this are by changing all dairy choices to low-fat varieties and by baking or broiling foods rather than frying them.

Types of Fat and Sources

Monounsaturated Fats
- Canola oil
- Olive oil
- Olives
- Avocados
- Almonds
- Cashews
- Pecans
- Peanuts
- Sesame seeds

Polyunsaturated Fats
- Corn oil
- Safflower oil
- Soybean oil
- Sunflower seeds
- Walnuts

Saturated Fats
- Bacon
- Butter
- Cheese
- Coconut
- Cream
- Lard
- Palm oil
- Solid vegetable shortening

Note: Most foods contain a mixture of fats from all three categories. For example, butter is 62 percent saturated fat, 4 percent polyunsaturated fat and 29 percent monounsaturated fat. By comparison, olive oil is only 14 percent saturated fat, 8 percent polyunsaturated fat and 74 percent monounsaturated fat.

Getting "enough" monounsaturated fat in the diet in the form of olive oil may be just as important in reducing heart disease as keeping cholesterol and saturated fat consumption low.

The NHS findings indicated that high consumption of trans fats (see the "Trans Fats" box, page 21) increased a woman's risk of heart disease just as consumption of saturated fats did. Trans fats seem to increase the LDL, or "bad," cholesterol level, a risk factor for heart disease. The researchers speculated that among those whose fat intake has been very high, the risk of developing heart disease could be reduced by an impressive 53 percent simply by replacing just 2 percent of calories from trans fats with unsaturated fats! This could be achieved by replacing margarine and shortening with olive oil in cooking and avoiding processed convenience foods.

Researchers learned that the *type of fat* consumed may affect the *amount* of the fat that one may consume for the heart-protective benefit. Surprisingly, getting "enough" monounsaturated fat in the diet in the form of olive oil may be just as important in reducing heart disease as keeping cholesterol and saturated fat consumption low. Cutting back on the consumption of animal products is not the only

Types of Fat and Their Effect on Cholesterol

Monounsaturated Fat: Reduces serum (blood) amounts of LDL ("bad," or "lousy," cholesterol) and increases levels of HDL ("good" cholesterol).
Polyunsaturated Fat: Reduces serum (blood) amounts of LDL but does not increase levels of HDL.
Saturated Fat: Increases serum (blood) amounts of LDL.

Note: Physical activity can also create a favorable blood-fat profile, with increased HDL and lower LDL and triglycerides.

way to reduce low-density lipoprotein (LDL) levels in the blood and help prevent heart disease, researchers believe. Maintaining high blood-serum levels of high-density lipoproteins (HDL) may be just as important in preventing heart disease.

The levels of different types of cholesterol—HDL, LDL, and trigylcerides—in the bloodstream depend largely on diet. For most of us, cholesterol levels are directly related to what we put on our

Trans Fats

In nature, fatty acids exist in a certain chemical form, called the "cis" form. Fats are changed from the cis to the trans form when oils, which are mostly polyunsaturated fats, have hydrogen added to them in a process called hydrogenation. The hydrogenation process makes liquid oils solid at room temperature. This process became popular in the late 1960s, when polyunsaturated margarine began to replace butter in our diet. (Polyunsaturated fats are formed with several double bonds, or spaces, in their chemical chain. These spaces can accept hydrogen molecules in the hydrogenation process. In completely saturated fats, all the spaces are filled, so they are called "saturated.")

Margarine and vegetable shortening are examples of products formed by hydrogenation. Eating fats that are saturated by hydrogenation appears to increase one's risk of developing heart disease even more than eating natural saturated fats does, because of the trans fats that are formed. (Some people use butter rather than margarine for this reason–but an even better choice would be to substitute olive oil.) Trans fats increase the "lousy" LDL cholesterol and may decrease the "good" HDL levels.

At present, labels do not indicate the presence of trans fats in food products, but that may change in the near future. Manufacturers are being made aware of the need for this information, and some are listing this information even before the law mandates it. Commercial baked goods–including pastries, cookies, and crackers–are commonly high in hydrogenated fats and therefore trans fats. Read labels on these foods and choose carefully; better yet, avoid them and make your own baked goods using oil rather than butter or margarine if you can.

plates. Eating a diet low in cholesterol and saturated fat (found in animal products) does reduce LDL levels in the blood, but, on the other hand, it does not raise HDL levels (the "good" cholesterol). Research from Penn State University recently showed that replacing saturated and polyunsaturated fat (found in soybean and corn oil) intake with monounsaturated fat (found in olive oil and nuts) can raise HDL levels as well as prevent a troublesome rise in triglyceride levels associated with low-fat diets. Triglyceride levels are commonly noted to go up in diets that are significantly restricted in fat, especially if simple sugars replace the fat calories normally consumed. Use the table above to help you choose fats wisely as part of eating the Mediterranean way.

Antioxidants

Antioxidants are important allies in maintaining good health because they protect cells from damage by free radicals. Free radicals are natural, necessary molecules that circulate in the body in order to attack and defeat infection and destroy unwanted bacteria through a process called oxidation. (See the "Cholesterol and Triglycerides" box, page 16, for more information about free radicals.) When too many free radicals are present in the body, however, they can damage cells and contribute to the aging process, heart disease, and cancer.

Antioxidants block the oxidation process, protecting LDL and reducing the buildup of arterial plaque. Reducing LDL levels is one way of decreasing oxidation; consuming plant foods high in antioxidants is another. High levels of antioxidants in the Mediterranean diet are responsible in part for the decreased risk of heart disease observed in this region, but they play a more significant role in the prevention of other diseases, specifically cancer.

↑ Antioxidants = ↓ oxidation of LDL = ↓ decreased formation of plaques = ↓ decreased heart disease

Much of the protective effect of the Mediterranean diet against disease is related to the high consumption of fruits and vegetables, which are good sources of antioxidants such as carotenoids and vitamins C and E. The protective effect of diet on cancer in particular is related to eating foods high in antioxidants and other protective phytochemicals (*phyto* = plant), which are most abundant in primarily plant-based eating plans. The precise mechanisms of cancer development have not been defined yet. Strong evidence suggests that oxidation (the same process that leads to arterial plaque and heart disease) plays an important role.

People often assume that if consuming antioxidants in the diet is healthful, then taking antioxidant supplements in quantity must be even better. This hasn't been proved, however. Where vitamin E is concerned, a supplement may be required in order to consume amounts large enough to reduce heart disease. Carotenoids, found in

Antioxidants: Dietary Sources and Benefits

Antioxidant	Vegetables	Fruit	Health Benefits
Carotenoids (for example, beta-carotene, lycopene)	Carrots, sweet potatoes, broccoli, winter squash, romaine lettuce	Apricots, cantaloupe, papayas, peaches	Improves immunity; antioxidant
Vitamin C	Broccoli, Brussels sprouts, cabbage, cauliflower, tomatoes, green peppers, potatoes	Citrus (oranges, grapefruit), straw-berries, cantaloupe	May reduce heart disease and some cancers; improves immunity
Vitamin E	Dark-green, leafy vegetables (broccoli, spinach, romaine lettuce)	Apples, apricots, nectarines, peaches	Improves immunity and protects against heart disease

fruits and vegetables, may reduce cancer risk. More than 400 carotenoids are found naturally in plant foods; beta-carotene is the most familiar example of this type of phytochemical. In one study of lung cancer patients, however, beta-carotene supplements actually *increased* mortality.

The best way to get all the nutrients you need is by eating a diet rich in a variety of plant foods. If you feel you absolutely cannot increase your plant food consumption sufficiently, try a multivitamin complex and avoid excessively high doses of any nutrient.

Fiber and Health

The Mediterranean diet is high in soluble and insoluble fiber. Insoluble fiber comes from fruits, vegetables, whole grains, seeds, and nuts that are part of the daily diet. Legumes, which are also an important protein source around the Mediterranean, provide much of the soluble fiber.

> The best way to get all the nutrients you need is by eating a diet rich in a variety of plant foods.

Soluble fiber helps reduce blood cholesterol levels. Soluble fiber decreases both total blood cholesterol and low-density lipoprotein (LDL) cholesterol. High levels of LDL cholesterol are a risk factor for heart disease. Soluble fiber appears to work by reducing the body's reabsorption of cholesterol-containing bile acids from the small intestine. This cholesterol is then replaced from liver stores, reducing the overall amount in the body.

Soluble fiber controls the increase in blood glucose following a meal, which is helpful in controlling blood-glucose levels in those with diabetes. It is thought that the fiber dissolves and slows stomach emptying, spreading the absorption of the glucose over a longer period of time.

High-fiber diets have also been shown to reduce cancer in groups of people, decreasing breast, prostate, colon, and rectal cancer risk. Fiber gives form, bulk, and thickness to plants. Soluble and insoluble fiber aids digestion, keeping wastes moving along the digestive tract. This is an important contribution, because it limits the time your intestinal wall is exposed to carcinogens in the diet. Consuming fiber also makes stools bulkier, binding and diluting carcinogens that may be present. Fiber is found only in plant foods, such as whole grains, fruits, and vegetables—another example of how following a plant-based diet can keep you healthy.

The recommended intake for fiber is 25 to 30 grams per day. That probably sounds like a lot, given that the average American consumes only 11 grams per day. However, if you eat five servings of fruits and vegetables each day, along with whole-grain breads and cereals, you are well on your way to achieving your target consumption rate. Refer to the table "High-Fiber Foods" below for the fiber content of some common foods.

Complex Carbohydrates and Disease Prevention. Beans, grains, pasta, bread, and the starchy vegetables are the best sources of complex carbohydrates. These foods are good sources of energy, B vitamins, minerals, and fiber. Most sources are also low in cholesterol and saturated fat—good for heart-disease prevention. Because the Mediterranean diet is naturally high in complex carbohydrates and low in sodium and simple sugars, it is a flavorful

High-Fiber Foods

Food	Serving Size	Grams of fiber
Apples	1 medium	4
Beans (black, pinto, red)	1/2 cup	7
Broccoli	1/2 cup	3
Brown rice	1/2 cup	3
Carrots	1/2 cup	2
Green peas	1/2 cup	4
Lentils	1/2 cup	8
Pears	1 medium	3
Berries	1/2 cup	3–4
Whole-grain bread	1 slice	2–5

and healthful eating plan that can be easily modified to fit the needs of people with diabetes as well as those concerned about preventing heart disease. When the diet is combined with regular exercise, desirable weight and blood-glucose levels are also easier to manage. This factor is an important consideration because individuals with diabetes are at higher risk for developing heart disease and encounter other health complications if the blood-glucose levels are not controlled.

Mediterranean Heart Diet
Sample Menu for Women

Breakfast
2 slices whole-wheat toast with 2 tablespoons jam
or
1/2 cup cooked oatmeal with 2 tablespoons raisins and 1/2 cup fat-free milk
and
1/2 cup chopped fresh fruit with 1/4 cup plain fat-free yogurt
Coffee or tea

Lunch
2 cups vegetable or lentil soup
4 or 5 whole-wheat crackers
1 ounce cheese or 1 ounce nuts
1 apple or peach

Dinner
2 to 3 cups pasta, beans, and vegetables and 1 tablespoon freshly grated Parmesan cheese
or
2 to 3 ounces grilled fish with herb-and-crumb topping
1/2 cup cooked rice or couscous
1/2 cup cooked, chopped broccoli with fresh lemon juice
and
2 cups mixed greens salad with tomatoes and carrots
2 tablespoons salad dressing made with olive oil
5 ounces wine (optional)
1 cup mixed berries topped with 1/4 cup vanilla fat-free yogurt

Good Health Equals Diet Plus Lifestyle

Although diet plays a central role in maintaining good health, it is not the only element to consider when making a commitment to healthful living. Genetic factors and environmental exposures play important roles also. While inheriting a genetic predisposition to a disease is beyond our individual control, we can adopt healthful habits that may prevent or significantly delay these diseases from developing. The following suggestions can help.

Maintain a healthy weight. Overweight and obesity are risk factors for many diseases, including heart disease. If you are

Mediterranean Heart Diet Sample Menu for Men

Breakfast

1/2 cup cooked oatmeal with 2 tablespoons raisins and 1/2 cup fat-free milk
2 slices whole-wheat toast with 2 tablespoons jam
1/2 to 1 cup chopped fresh fruit
Coffee or tea

Lunch

3 cups vegetable or lentil soup
6 to 8 whole-wheat crackers
1 ounce cheese or 1 ounce nuts
1 apple or peach

Dinner

3 to 4 cups pasta, beans, and vegetables and 2 tablespoons freshly grated Parmesan cheese
or
4 to 5 ounces grilled fish with herb-and-crumb topping
1 cup cooked rice or couscous
3/4 cup cooked chopped broccoli with fresh lemon juice
and
2 cups mixed greens salad with tomatoes and carrots
2 to 3 tablespoons salad dressing made with olive oil
5 to 10 ounces wine (optional)
1 cup mixed berries with 1/4 cup vanilla fat-free yogurt

overweight and you would like to lose weight, you need to reduce your total energy intake. The Mediterranean diet can provide a safe, well-rounded, satisfying, and nutritious way to take that step toward lifelong weight loss. Sample menu plans for men and women are provided in the boxes on pages 26 and 27.

If you smoke, stop! Smoking is strongly associated with lung cancer and increases one's risk of developing heart disease, high blood pressure, and other cancers.

Get regular checkups. Many cancers, heart disease, and other health problems can be eliminated or their effect minimized if detected early.

Get enough sleep, and relax. Regular sleep and stress reduction can reduce your risk for disease and simply make you feel better.

Get moving! Physical activity is an effective, natural way of relieving stress and promoting good sleep, and it provides many other health benefits, which are discussed next.

Physical Activity. The reduced rates of cancer and heart disease seen in the Seven Countries Study and other studies are largely due to diet but are in part also related to the higher level of physical activity in the Mediterranean region. In North America, we tend to think of exercise as something we "do." Some of us have exercise routines that we follow religiously; others don't make exercise a regular part of the day. Most of us don't incorporate the easiest ways of exercising: For example, we don't take the stairs at work, and we don't walk or ride our bikes to the local market—we automatically choose to take the elevator or drive the car instead. We see routine activities like these as time-consuming hassles, even though some of us are willing to use up much more energy and time on a Stairmaster or treadmill.

The Mediterranean approach to exercise is to incorporate fitness into everyday activities. Most people in that region walk to the markets, walk home carrying their purchases, and walk to a nearby home for a social gathering. Family outings often include hiking, swimming, and bike riding. These activities are not perceived as exercise, yet they certainly contribute to the overall health of the people in the Mediterranean. Perceiving exercise as an everyday part of life makes sticking with an active lifestyle easier. We provide exercise tips to help you get started on a fitness program on page 47.

Important: Check with your physician before starting any type of exercise program.

Finding Balance in the Mediterranean Diet

Two Food Pyramids: How Do They Compare?

A look at the U.S. Department of Agriculture (USDA) food guide pyramid, the one most of us are familiar with, shows that Americans today are encouraged to consume the same kinds of foods that the Mediterranean peoples enjoy—fruits, vegetables, whole grains, limited meat and dairy—yet in very different proportions in the daily diet. Evidence suggests that it is the emphasis on certain foods (fruits, vegetables, olive oil, and whole grains) in the Mediterranean diet that is important.

The Mediterranean diet pyramid was designed by Oldways Preservation and Exchange Trust to reflect graphically the types of food consumed as part of the healthful Mediterranean lifestyle. The Mediterranean diet pyramid does not specify serving sizes because the proportions will vary depending on the area of the Mediterranean under discussion. Instead, this pyramid conveys an overall picture of the foods that make up this healthful diet.

The USDA food guide pyramid is not based on established dietary practices that Americans follow routinely. The pyramid was designed by scientists to help improve a national eating pattern that has been responsible in part for increasing rates of chronic diseases, including heart disease and cancer. It is based on well-documented research. Unlike the Mediterranean diet pyramid, the USDA food guide pyramid makes specific recommendations as to the number of servings to consume of each food group each day. (Compare the two pyramids on pages 30 and 31.)

The essential difference between the two pyramids is that the USDA food guide pyramid has never been tested in a population, whereas the Mediterranean diet has been followed by thousands of people for hundreds of years. The Mediterranean pyramid represents all the foods that are emphasized in the traditional Mediterranean diet. The people of this region who ate this way have consistently experienced lower rates of chronic disease and longer adult life expectancies.

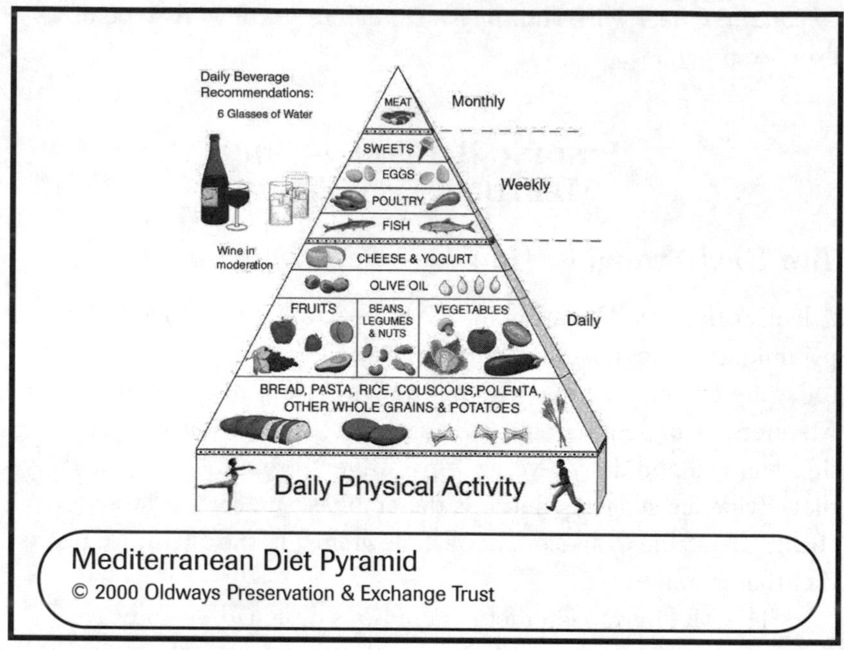

Mediterranean Diet Pyramid
© 2000 Oldways Preservation & Exchange Trust

Food from Plant Sources

In the Mediterranean, fruits, vegetables, nuts, beans, legumes, whole grains, seeds, and olives are the heart of the diet. Diets like this one that are high in plant foods are also high in complex carbohydrates, fiber, vitamins, antioxidants, and phytochemicals (see below). Phytochemicals—chemicals found in plants—appear to have numerous health benefits. Scientists believe we have discovered only a fraction of these benefits, with many more to be discovered in the future.

Fruits and Vegetables. Known health benefits of consuming lots of fruits and vegetables in the diet include reduced heart disease and cancer risk and the promotion of weight loss. Antioxidants in the body, supplied through the consumption of fruits and vegetables, reduce the risk of several diseases. Cruciferous vegetables, such as broccoli and cabbage, have been shown to reduce the risk of breast, lung, gastrointestinal, and other cancers. Fruits and vegetables are good sources of vitamins C and E, as well as carotenoids, all beneficial to health. Refer to the table on page 23 to learn which foods are high in these health-promoting nutrients.

One piece of fruit or one vegetable contains as many as 20 different nutrients and 100 different phytochemicals. Clearly, these

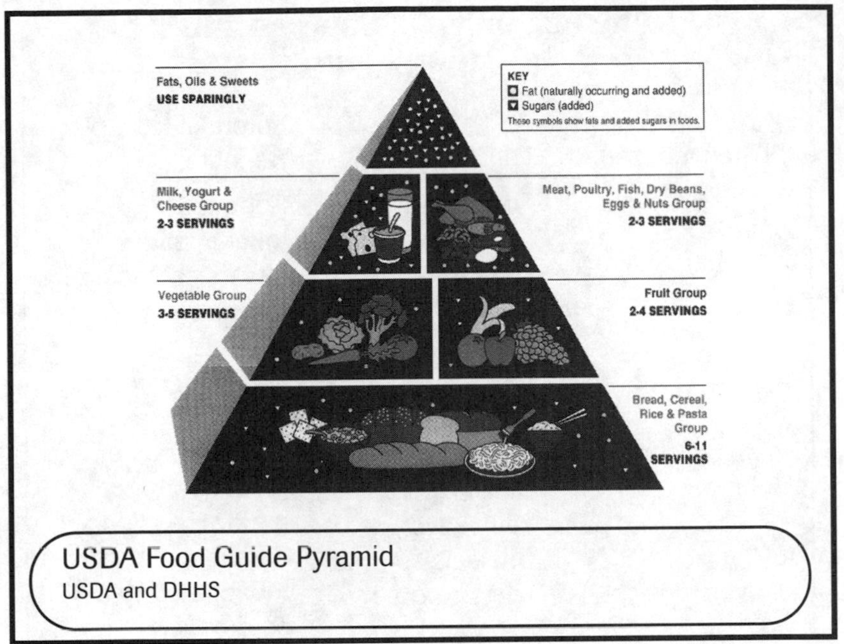

USDA Food Guide Pyramid
USDA and DHHS

foods are nutritional powerhouses, with benefits to our health that we may not even know yet. It appears that these elements need to work together to provide the greatest health benefit. For this reason, supplements do not supply the same health benefits as the whole food. In fact, research using isolated phytochemicals such as beta-carotene has actually shown an *increase* in cancer rates. The lesson is this: Consume the whole food rather than isolated phytochemicals to achieve the health-promoting "synergy" that only real food can provide, partly because we don't know whether some of the actions are caused by one phytochemical or by a group of them working together. To give you an idea of how many phytochemicals our foods contain and the benefits we know of so far, refer to the table below, which identifies a few that have been well studied and their possible health benefits.

Grains. Whole grains are emphasized in both the Mediterranean diet and the diet suggested by the USDA food guide pyramid. Whole grains are a major source of daily calories and complex carbohydrates. Breads, cereals, rice, and pasta are all made from grains. Whole grains are high in B vitamins, folate, and fiber.

High in energy and low in fat, these foods are good candidates for healthful eating. They do contribute significantly to total calorie intake, however. Consume them in moderation to maintain a

Phytochemicals: Sources and Health Benefits

Phytochemical(s)	Food	Potential Health Benefits
Alpha-linolenic acid	Flaxseed, walnuts	Reduces inflammation, lowers cholesterol, may protect against breast cancer, improves immunity
Isothiocyanates: Sulforaphane	Broccoli, kale, radish, cabbage, cauliflower, Brussels sprouts, mustard greens	Reduces risk of tobacco-induced tumors by reducing damage to cells by tobacco-related carcinogens
Indoles	Cabbage, broccoli, Brussels sprouts, watercress, cauliflower, turnips, kohlrabi, kale, rutabaga, horseradish, mustard greens	May protect against hormone-related cancers by inactivating estrogen, inhibits growth of cancer cells
Quercetin	Pear skin, apple skin, bell pepper, kohlrabi, tomato leaves, onion, wine, grape juice	Associated with reduced coronary heart disease, antioxidant, inhibits blood clotting
Monoterpene: Limonene	Citrus (peel, membrane), mint, caraway, thyme	Antioxidant, reduces risk of skin and breast cancer, induces cancer-cell death, reduces cholesterol and premenstrual symptoms

Phytochemical(s)	Food	Potential Health Benefits
Organosulfur compounds: Allylic acid	Garlic, onions, watercress, cruciferous vegetables, thyme, scallions	Reduces risk of gastric, colon, and lung cancer; prevents blood clotting in arteries; reduces cholesterol, blood pressure; protects gut from harmful bacteria
Carotenoids: Beta-carotene, alpha-carotene, lutein, lycopene	Yellow, orange, and dark vegetables	Reduces risk of cataracts, coronary artery disease, lung and breast cancers, enhances immunity in the elderly
Curcumin	Turmeric	May lower cholesterol, reduces skin-cancer risk
Flavonols, polyphenols: Catechins	Green and black tea, berries	Reduces risk of gastric cancer, antioxidant, protects against chemically induced cancers and skin cancer
Lycopene	Tomatoes, tomato sauce, catsup, guava, dried apricots, watermelon	Antioxidant, may reduce risk of prostate cancer and cardiovascular disease
Lignans	High-fiber foods, especially seeds	Reduces cancer risk (colon), reduces cholesterol levels
Polyacetylene	Parsley, carrots, celery	Decreases risk of tobacco-induced tumors

continues

Phytochemical(s)	Food	Potential Health Benefits
Phenolic acids	Cruciferous vegetables, eggplant, peppers, tomatoes, celery, parsley, soy, licorice root, flaxseed, citrus, whole grains, berries	Reduces lung- and skin-cancer risk
Tannins	Blueberries and cranberries	Prevents urinary-tract infection by blocking bacterial growth
Resveratrol	Red wine, grapes	Cardio-protective: inhibits cells in blood from clogging arteries; anti-tumor capacity
Cynarin	Artichokes	Decreases cholesterol levels
Ellagic acid	Wine, grapes, currants, nuts (pecans), berries (strawberries, blackberries, raspberries), seeds	Reduces cancer risk, reduces LDL while increasing HDL cholesterol levels

healthful body weight. When consumed in appropriate portions, complex carbohydrates may actually promote weight loss. Try some of the grains suggested in the box on page 35—some of them may be new to you.

Beans and Legumes. Like whole grains, beans and legumes are an excellent source of fiber in the Mediterranean diet. Beans, legumes, and nuts are given special emphasis in the Mediterranean diet pyramid. This important food group provides a high percentage of protein in the Mediterranean diet, but it is of a significantly different type than the protein found in meat, poultry, and fish—the sources we tend to rely on for protein in North America. Beans and legumes contain complex carbohydrates, fiber, B vitamins, and a variety of other beneficial vitamins and minerals.

Because they are plant foods, beans and legumes contain no cholesterol or saturated fat, as meats do. Replacing most of the protein you get from animal sources with protein from plant sources not only reduces your intake of saturated fat and cholesterol but also adds fiber and nutrients—adding up to a noticeable improvement in your diet overall.

Fat Intake as Olive Oil. In many regions of the Mediterranean, fat intake exceeds 35 percent of total daily calories consumed. This is a high percentage compared to what many national health organizations in North America recommend. The difference can be attributed to the type of fats that are implied by the two pyramids. In the Mediterranean, most fat in the diet comes from olive oil, which has certain heart-healthy properties. In North America, most people get fat in their diets from a mixture of unsaturated *and* saturated fats (such as butter). Saturated fats, as we have seen, contribute to heart disease and should be limited in the diet. The USDA food guide pyramid focuses on *total* fat consumed; it does not distinguish among types of fat, hence the lower overall daily percentage of fat recommended in the USDA pyramid compared to that shown in the Mediterranean pyramid. In addition, most Americans do not have a healthy body weight; thus excess fat intake is likely to result in excess body fat—a pattern markedly different from that of Mediterranean people.

New Grains to Try

- Bulgur
- Wheat berry
- Brown rice
- Barley
- Quinoa (pronounced KEEN-wa)

Nuts. After olive oil, nuts supply a large percentage of the fat consumed in the Mediterranean diet. Nuts are a good source of protein and can replace animal protein sources in the diet. Unlike meats, nuts have no cholesterol and usually are low in saturated fat also. Some nuts are high in beneficial vitamin E and omega-3 fatty acids, which may protect against heart disease. Meat offers neither of these beneficial nutrients.

In the Mediterranean diet, nuts are used sparingly, because they are high in calories. They are used in cooking primarily as tasty accents. They are not consumed out of hand (for example, while watching football on TV!). Because of their fat content, nuts not only add texture and flavor to a meal but also help those who eat them to feel satisfied or "full." Nuts contain differing amounts of monounsaturated, polyunsaturated, and saturated fat depending on type. Avoid nuts that are high in saturated fat. Choose to eat them less frequently than their lower-fat counterparts. Refer to the table below for the fat content of nuts commonly consumed in the Mediterranean diet.

Red Wine. A small glass of wine is pictured alongside the Mediterranean diet pyramid but does not appear next to the USDA

Nuts

Type of Nut (1 ounce)	Monounsaturated Fat	Polyunsaturated Fat	Saturated Fat	Total Fat
Almonds	9.5 gm	3.1 gm	1.4 gm	14.7 gm
Cashews	7.8 gm	2.2 gm	2.6 gm	13.2 gm
Hazelnuts	13.9 gm	1.7 gm	1.3 gm	17.8 gm
Macadamia nuts	16.5 gm	0.4 gm	3.1 gm	20.9 gm
Peanuts	6.9 gm	4.4 gm	1.9 gm	14.0 gm
Pine nuts (pignoli)	6.5 gm	7.3 gm	2.7 gm	17.3 gm
Pistachios	9.3 gm	2.1 gm	1.7 gm	13.7 gm

gm = gram

food guide pyramid. People in Mediterranean cultures (with the exception of Islamic regions) traditionally enjoy a moderate amount of wine with meals, and wine plays an integral part in religious and cultural practices. No other type of alcoholic beverage is identified as part of the diet.

Recent scientific studies suggest that moderate wine consumption may increase high-density lipoproteins (HDL) levels in the bloodstream and help decrease the production of low-density lipoproteins (LDL). Wine may also help activate the body's natural anti-clotting enzyme, thus reducing the tendency of plaque formation along arterial walls. Wine is thought to reduce heart-disease risk through these mechanisms.

Moderate consumption is key, however! For women, that means about 1 drink a day (5 ounces of wine), and for men, 1 to 2 glasses of wine a day. Excessive alcohol intake is an extreme hazard to one's health. It can damage the brain, heart, liver, and pancreas, and it increases the risk of developing certain cancers.

For that reason, it is important that we adapt this aspect of the Mediterranean lifestyle carefully to our own traditions and social context. In our culture, alcohol is not consumed by adolescents and children, and it should not be consumed by those who are unable to limit themselves to only moderate amounts of alcohol. Drinking responsibly is always important. Pregnant women in particular should not drink alcohol at all. Some evidence suggests that moderate alcohol intake may increase the risk of breast cancer, and women at risk for breast cancer should probably avoid alcohol altogether. Although there are health benefits to moderate alcohol intake, it is important that you decide what level, if any, is compatible with your lifestyle and then act responsibly. Discuss this matter with your health-care provider if you are uncertain about the potential risk or benefit in your own case.

Foods from Animal Sources

North Americans typically consume meat and dairy products in significantly higher quantities than do people in the Mediterranean. (Answer quickly: How often did you eat fast food in the form of meaty sandwiches and milkshakes in the past week? Did you add milk to your coffee every time you poured a cup?) Protein in the Mediterranean diet, on the other hand, is derived largely from beans, legumes, and nuts. The USDA food guide pyramid recommends 5 to 6 servings of meat and dairy per day, equally divided between the two sources. In the traditional Mediterranean diet, animal products of *any* type were consumed in small amounts, about three servings total a day, mostly in the form of cheese and yogurt. Fish and poultry were consumed more often than red meat, but still in small, infrequent servings. Fish is important to the diet in some areas of the Mediterranean, but it is not consumed uniformly throughout the region. Red meat is the least emphasized food, as the Mediterranean diet pyramid shows.

Red Meat, Poultry, and Fish. Protein is an essential part of any diet, but most North Americans eat too much of it at the expense of consuming more complex carbohydrates, fresh fruits, and vegetables. The average adult only needs 50 to 60 grams of protein a day; most Americans consume twice that amount. The USDA food guide pyramid recommends getting most dietary protein from animal sources. Many people wrongly believe this is the only source of "real" protein. We know that animal sources of protein are high in cholesterol and often high in saturated fat, the overconsumption of which contributes to heart-disease risk. In the areas of the world where red meat is consumed less frequently, cancer rates are lower.

Current research suggests that consuming less protein each day and increasing plant and whole-grain protein sources yield better health benefits. Fish, beans, nuts, and whole grains have been identified as better sources of protein. Choose them over red meat and poultry most of the time.

In the traditional Mediterranean diet, all foods from animal sources were used sparingly. In 1960, the average person's consumption of animal protein in Crete was about 13 ounces a week. Originally, red meat was not readily available in the Mediterranean region. It was consumed rarely, once or twice a month, usually on a special occasion. Today, red meat consumption is rising, thanks to increasing economic prosperity in the region, but as a result, overall health in this population will certainly suffer. Meat is not an essential food; meat does not contain nutrients that cannot be obtained from other foods.

Recent research indicates that fish is the best source of animal protein.

Changing Patterns

The region that gave us such a healthful approach to eating is itself leaning toward a more sedentary lifestyle and a Westernized diet–that is, a diet higher in saturated fats and meat consumption and lower in fruits, vegetables, grains, and legumes. However, studies in the 1990s indicate that the rate of coronary heart disease in the Mediterranean is still lower than that of the United States.

In 1960, the people of the Mediterranean region consumed an average of 4.5 to 15 ounces of fish per week. Recent research indicates that fish is the best source of animal protein. The people of Japan currently have the longest life expectancy in the world, and they consume 19 to 24 ounces of fish per week. Most fish are lower in saturated fat than their animal counterparts, and several fish (primarily salmon, mackerel, anchovies, and tuna) are high in omega-3 fatty acids, which may reduce the risk of heart disease and stroke.

Dairy Foods. Dairy products do not make up a large percentage of what is consumed according to the Mediterranean diet pyramid, which is quite different from the 2 to 3 servings a day suggested by the USDA food guide pyramid. However, of all animal products consumed in the Mediterranean diet, yogurt and cheese—rather than meats and fish—are the mainstay. This emphasis has certain health advantages. Dairy products are a great source of calcium, which is necessary for maintaining healthy bones. An adequate amount of calcium in the diet decreases the risk of developing osteoporosis. It is difficult to get all the calcium you need through nondairy sources. To do so, you will probably need to take a calcium supplement and eat dark-green, leafy vegetables that are high in calcium every day, such as bok choy or Swiss chard.

At the time of the Seven Countries Study, low- and nonfat dairy products were not available. All dairy products were made from whole milk, so they contained a lot of fat. This didn't present a health problem, because Mediterranean peoples use cheese differently than Americans typically do. Rarely consumed by itself, cheese was used more often as a seasoning. It never made up a major part of any meal. Strong, flavorful cheese, such as Greek feta, might be used in small amounts for a big flavor impact. In the 1960s, the average person in Crete ate 3 ounces of cheese and 1 cup (8 ounces) of dairy per day, usually in the form of yogurt rather than milk.

Low-fat cheeses and yogurt are now produced in abundance. These are good options if you wish to consume 2 to 3 servings of dairy per day. If you intend to cut down on your daily dairy intake and want to reduce it to 1 or 2 servings per day, you may want to consider small amounts of full-fat dairy options, especially flavorful cheeses. Cheese can lose a lot of flavor and texture when made low-fat. Using a low-fat cheese might encourage you to use more of it than you would a full-fat cheese, canceling the benefit.

Practical Pointers for Changing Your Diet

It is difficult to slow down, prepare, and eat a healthful diet in our rush-rush world. We grab a doughnut on the way to work and maybe a deli sandwich, heavy on the meat, at lunch. In this section, we'll show you easy ways to incorporate Mediterranean-diet concepts into your lifestyle for better health overall. We'll tell you how to shop, what foods to avoid, and ways to stick with the Mediterranean lifestyle while you're on the go.

The Food

It's time to put the principles of the Mediterranean heart diet into practice. To follow a Mediterranean eating plan, make plant foods the focus of your dishes. Most of the food you see on your plate should come from vegetables, fruits, legumes, and grains. Add nuts and olive oil for flavor and texture. Use yogurt often; it makes a terrific base for all kinds of good-tasting sauces and dressings. Consume small amounts of hard cheeses with meals to add flavor, perhaps grated over pasta or sprinkled lightly over a medley of colorful steamed vegetables. Prepare meals with meat only a few times a week, and when possible, choose fish over poultry or red meat at those times.

Shopping. You are about to embark on an exciting new experience; you will discover new flavors and textures in just a few pages. To transform your refrigerator and pantry into a Mediterranean cooking zone, keep a few essentials on hand at all times. Shopping for these items doesn't have to be a chore; the box below can help. With these items in your cupboard, you will always be able to prepare a healthful, delicious meal in a short amount of time.

You may have to hunt for a few of the suggested ingredients if your local grocery store does not carry them. (You can always ask your grocery store to order the ingredients for you; many are happy to do so through their distributors.) Or you may take the opportunity to try some local specialty stores, such as a real Greek, Middle Eastern, or Italian deli. You will be amazed at the variety of foods available. Experiment with new olives, olive oils, and herbs. This is half the fun!

Be adventurous with new kinds of produce; try new fruits and vegetables and see how you like them. Shop at a farmer's market if you can; it is a fun way to buy delicious, fresh produce. You will find an amazing variety of fruits and vegetables in season. As you begin to cultivate a plant-based diet, you may want to change your usual shopping habits slightly. You may want to buy produce at least twice a week so that you always have fresh fruits and vegetables on hand. Keep a few cans or frozen packages of fruits or vegetables in the kitchen for those times when you feel short of time.

The Essentials

Dried and fresh herbs
Dried beans and lentils; canned beans and lentils, for quick meals
Full-flavored cheeses, such as Parmesan and feta
High-quality vinegars, such as balsamic
Olive oils (extra-light and extra-virgin)
Olives
Nuts
Pasta, several shapes for variety
Fresh, seasonal fruits, such as melons, citrus, and berries
Fresh, seasonal vegetables, particularly dark-green types
Frozen vegetables, a variety to use when you just can't get to the market
Whole grains, such as bulgur and brown rice
Whole-grain breads
Yogurt (low-fat or nonfat)

Eating Out

Eating out at restaurants or friends' homes can wreak havoc on any healthful eating plan. Try these tips to help you follow a Mediterranean-style eating plan away from home:

Avoid creamy sauces. Sauces made with cream are high in saturated fat. Instead try to find an oil-based sauce, or choose a dish that is accompanied by a fruit salsa or a tomato-and-herb sauce.

Order a dish with lots of vegetables. Salads are usually a good option when eating out. Be careful of the dressing you use and how much. Dressings in restaurants are often the full-fat variety and are likely to be high in saturated fat. Ask for low-fat dressing, vinaigrette, or olive oil and extra seasoning. To avoid salads that are coated in dressing, ask for the dressing on the side so you can add the amount you want. Some people find that dipping a fork into the dressing and then spearing a bit of salad to eat provides maximum flavor and uses minimal amounts of the salad dressing.

Try fish varieties that are new to you. Try fish in a restaurant setting if you find preparing fish at home to be somewhat tricky. Avoid creamy casserole dishes and opt instead for grilled selections.

Don't empty the bread basket and then eat the full meal that follows if you are watching calories. Eat "free" foods with mindfulness. It's easy to eat these foods without thinking, and pretty soon half a loaf of bread has disappeared. Decide when you sit down how much you will eat of it, then stick to your plan.

This is a great time to use olive oil on your bread instead of butter. If it isn't already on the table, ask your waiter to bring some. When you are having bread, request whole-grain varieties.

Split meals. Meals in restaurants are often two to three times the size of what we would eat at home. Split a meal with a friend or simply divide the meal in half and assume you will take the rest home. You can also request half portions when you order; many restaurants will oblige.

Eat slowly. It is common to eat meals so quickly that our bodies aren't given a chance to feel full. Enjoy your meal—slow down and savor it. Relax; talk with your dining companions.

Ask for fruit or vegetables to replace potatoes as a side to the main dish. Many restaurants are offering these sides as a standard option, but ask even if they aren't offered automatically.

Choose a salad, soup, or appetizer, or a combination of these, for your meal instead of a large entrée. You'll save money and still eat very well.

Try new foods. Go off the beaten path and try local ethnic restaurants to broaden your enjoyment of all kinds of produce, fish, grains, and beans.

The Mediterranean Lifestyle

The more successful we are in our working lives, the less time we seem to have to focus on ourselves and our family. We neglect our bodies and become less physically active. This is an important characteristic of American culture that contributes to our declining standard of health. In the Mediterranean, staying active, relaxing,

Snacking Tips

- Keep dried fruits in your desk drawer for a healthful energy boost at work.
- Keep a fruit basket or bowl on your kitchen counter or in your office, where you can reach it easily.
- Keep washed and cut vegetables in small bags in your refrigerator for an easy snack or quick "pick-up meal" when you're heading out the door.
- Try a vegetable juice mixture at your local juice bar.
- Make a fruit smoothie by blending fresh fruits, low-fat yogurt, and nonfat milk to a milkshake-like consistency in your blender. Add ice to the mixture for a hot-weather treat.
- Try a fruit pizza for dessert. On a dessert plate, cover a thin layer of low-fat yogurt with a variety of sliced fruits–orange, mango, berries, kiwi, and banana.
- Make an open-face sandwich: Layer a thin slice of fresh mozzarella with sliced tomatoes and basil on French bread.
- Prepare large batches of soups or salads and refrigerate or freeze leftovers to snack on later.
- For a filling, high-fiber snack or appetizer, try hummus on whole-grain bread, topped with tomato, cucumber, and onion.

enjoying time with family, and appreciating good food are all considered important to a successful life, and indeed these elements do contribute to good health. It is unrealistic to assume that we in North America can adopt a way of life that has evolved in a different culture, with a different economy, geography, and climate. But we can adopt some of the principles of this healthful lifestyle as our own. The next section suggests practical, easy ways to get started.

Suggestions for Enjoying the Mediterranean Lifestyle

Buy the best and freshest ingredients that you can find and afford. The better the quality of the food, the better you will like it. It will taste better and have more health-promoting nutrients. Try different kinds of olive oils, vinegars, and pasta. Start an herb garden (even in a window box), or plant a vegetable garden if you have the space. Seek out farmer's markets and buy vegetables and fruits in season for best flavor and texture.

Replace saturated fats such as butter, margarine, and shortening with olive oil in cooking and salad dressings and at the table. The object is to replace the type of fat, *not* to add additional sources of fat.

Add whole-grain breads to meals. Bake your own, or find a neighborhood bakery that sells good bread.

Eat less meat and poultry. Try to limit meat consumption to no more than 4 ounces a day, a few times per week. Use meat as a small part of a dish rather than as the main event.

Eat more fish. If fresh fish is not available, check out the frozen fish in your market. Newer methods of processing fish at sea can make frozen fish taste fresher than the "fresh" variety. Stay away from heavily processed frozen-fish products, such as fish sticks—choose plain filets that have been flash frozen and season them yourself.

Eat more dried beans and lentils. Add beans and lentils to soups, salads, and side dishes and feature them in main dishes. Seek out varieties of beans that are new to you. If you are short on time, use one of the many kinds of canned beans that are available.

Eat more salads and soups. Serve salads as a first course, with the main course, or after it. Try mixing in heartier greens, such as arugula and radicchio, to complement your usual lettuces. Like salad, a broth-based soup makes a good first course; it can take the edge off hunger and slow the pace of the meal. A hearty soup is always a popular main course, served with bread and a salad.

Serve more vegetables (and not just the usual ones). Try at least one new vegetable a week to introduce yourself to the bounty that is available. Serve vegetables in medleys you create, or serve two or three separate vegetable dishes at each meal.

Serve a glass of wine with food as the Europeans do, if you already enjoy wine. If you choose to drink wine, do so in moderation. Alcohol presents health risks for some people; check with your doctor before adding a glass of wine to your diet if you do not already drink wine.

Limit most desserts to special occasions. Choosing a piece of fruit instead makes it easy to increase the nutrients in your daily diet while also offering you a guilt-free treat. Try new varieties of fruits when you see them in the market; you might discover a new favorite.

Share at least one meal a day with family or friends. Too often we rush through the little time we have to spend with our family and friends. In the Mediterranean, spending time with family is a priority and is often centered around a meal. One meal may consist of many small courses and take hours to complete. Preparation of the meal is equally important and can be a fun activity for the whole family. Most of us do not have the hours to spend on enjoying our meals that the people of the Mediterranean have traditionally spent, but if we adjust our schedules a little, we can find a little more time for relaxing and enjoying food and family. Start slowly, simply by planning on having dinner as a family. Aim to eventually gather the whole family in the kitchen and get everyone involved in preparing the meals at least once or twice a week.

Stay physically fit. See page 47 for ways to keep fit and reduce stress.

You're on Your Way!

Now is your chance to join a tradition of healthful eating and living that has given the people of the Mediterranean long, healthful lives. You've seen that the Mediterranean diet is an easy, delicious, and satisfying way to reduce your risk of chronic disease. It is a lifestyle that the whole family can enjoy.

The rest of this book contains nutritious recipes that will tempt even the choosiest person in your family while promoting better health for everyone. We believe these recipes are so delightful that you will not have any trouble adopting a Mediterranean eating plan! Reread this section periodically for encouragement while making the change to a more healthful, active life. Best wishes for a healthy, invigorating, and more simplified lifestyle!

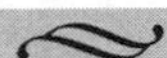

Get Moving!

- Take the stairs. Think of how many times you take the elevator at work or in department stores or malls. For every ten minutes you spend climbing stairs, you burn about 150 calories.
- Park farther away. When you go to the supermarket, office, or mall, don't park as close to the entrance as you can. Unless you have a physical ailment that limits your mobility, a short walk won't hurt. You might find it's more pleasant to avoid the parking congestion that develops close to the entrances of buildings.
- Walk or ride a bike. Weather and road conditions permitting, walking and bike riding are great ways to get where you are going and get some exercise. If you walk two miles, you will burn 160 calories.
- Join a gym. For those of us who live in icy, rainy, or very warm climates, outdoor activity may not always be an option. Joining a gym can be a great way to get physically active. Pick a gym that offers a variety of classes and has a swimming pool to keep you active.
- Take a hike. Make physical activity something you enjoy with family or friends on your days off. Movies are nice, but hiking and camping are great ways to enjoy the outdoors and spend time with loved ones.
- If you must watch TV, make a habit of exercising during commercials. Do sit-ups, push-ups, jump rope, or get on the treadmill–you can even challenge other family members!
- Find a friend you don't get to see often enough and begin meeting each morning to share a short walk. You'll get more exercise and gain precious time for catching up with each other.
- Avoid exercise burnout. Try a variety of exercise options. If you usually work out in a gym, change the routine every now and then by exercising outdoors instead, perhaps by taking a hike or riding a bicycle.
- Give your body the fuel it needs to be active. Don't exercise on an empty stomach. You will feel weak and soon run out of energy. East something small and high in carbohydrates about two hours before exercising (half a bagel, a piece of fruit, or nonfat yogurt are all good choices).

continues

- Drink lots of water! Exercising easily leads to dehydration if you don't drink water before, during, and after the activity. If you get thirsty, you are already dehydrated. Staying hydrated throughout the day decreases the likelihood that you will become dehydrated during exercise. Keep a bottle of water at work and sip it throughout the day.
- If you haven't already, you may want to incorporate weight-bearing exercises (such as push-ups, sit-ups, leg lifts) into your routine. Weight-bearing exercises build muscle and help increase your metabolism (which means you'll burn more calories). They strengthen bones, too.
- Don't be hard on yourself as you get started. Starting anything new takes time and effort. Set realistic goals with your doctor's help, especially if exercise is something you are just starting to add to your daily routine. Start with just ten minutes of walking a day, then slowly increase the time you spend at this activity to build intensity. From walking, move on to other activities and exercise you might enjoy.
- Set personal goals and monitor your success.
- Which exercise is best? The answer is, the one(s) you enjoy! Building physical activity into your life should be fun, not a chore—try new approaches until you find the one that works for you.

Easy-to-Prepare Recipes for the Mediterranean Diet

Nutritional Analysis

Nutrient analysis was calculated using the *Food Processor© for Windows Nutrition Analysis and Fitness* software program, version 7.4, copyright © 1987–1999 by ESHA Research. Analysis does not include optional ingredients. Only the primary choice is calculated. The first number provided for the range of servings is used for the calculation.

Appetizers

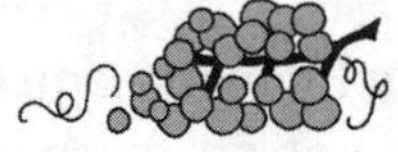

Beginning the meal with a light snack or starter is a good idea. It takes the edge off hunger and gives everyone a little time to unwind from the day's activities. Allow enough time to enjoy this pre-meal event. After all, dining should be a pleasant, unhurried occasion rather than a race to finish the meal. The people of the Mediterranean region know and practice this ritual daily; they enjoy each meal with family or friends as a celebrated social event.

Appetizers need not be fancy and should not be too filling. The idea is to whet the appetite, not to replace the meal to come.

For a dinner party, offer guests two or three different appetizers. Crackers, fresh vegetable sticks, or cheese can accompany most of the appetizers in this chapter. Bruschetta is a simple, crisp, herbed-enriched toast to serve alone or pair with a few nuts or olives. Anchovy Bruschetta is an example of a standard dish with a little extra embellishment that is easy to prepare—so the cook can enjoy being with the guests.

I like to share homegrown produce, especially cherry tomatoes, with friends. These delightful vegetables seem to be designed to be finger food. Fresh tomatoes are accented with a tangy tuna filling in Tuna-Stuffed Tomatoes. Caponata can also showcase the best and freshest produce, whether from your garden or the local farmer's market. Serve this vegetable medley either warm or cold.

An antipasto platter of cold marinated vegetables, sliced cold cuts, cheese, and even cold pasta dressed with vinaigrette is enticing. Keep serving sizes small, because the entrée is yet to come.

Avocado-Tomato Spread

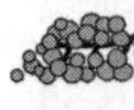

Mint adds a surprising flavor to this delicate avocado spread. Serve on toasted pita bread, bagels, or crackers. Avocado is a good source of monounsaturated fat.

1/2 cup Yogurt Cream Cheese, page 62
1/2 medium avocado, peeled, mashed
1 small tomato, seeded, chopped
1 teaspoon grated lemon zest
2 teaspoons fresh lemon juice
2 tablespoons pine nuts, chopped
2 teaspoons chopped fresh mint leaves

In a small bowl, thoroughly blend cream cheese and avocado. Stir in remaining ingredients. Cover and refrigerate until chilled. Makes 1 cup.

Each tablespoon contains:

Cal	Prot	Carb	Fib	Tot. Fat	Sat. Fat	Chol	Sodium
35	1g	2g	1g	3g	0g	0mg	18mg

Crab, Yogurt, and Olive Spread

Tangy, nutritious yogurt can be enjoyed by itself, embellished with herbs, or used as an ingredient in dishes like this. Serve this spread with toasted pita wedges or assorted vegetable sticks.

1/4 cup Yogurt Cream Cheese, page 62
2 tablespoons plain fat-free yogurt
2 tablespoons fat-free cottage cheese
2 teaspoons fresh lemon juice
2 tablespoons chopped pimiento
6 pitted green olives, chopped
1 teaspoon prepared horseradish
1 green onion, chopped
3 oz. cooked crabmeat, flaked
Dill weed, to taste

In a small bowl, blend Yogurt Cream Cheese with yogurt, cottage cheese, and lemon juice. Stir in remaining ingredients. Cover and refrigerate until ready to serve. Makes about 1 cup.

Each tablespoon contains:

Cal	Prot	Carb	Fib	Tot. Fat	Sat. Fat	Chol	Sodium
12	2g	1g	0g	0g	0g	4mg	66mg

Bruschetta

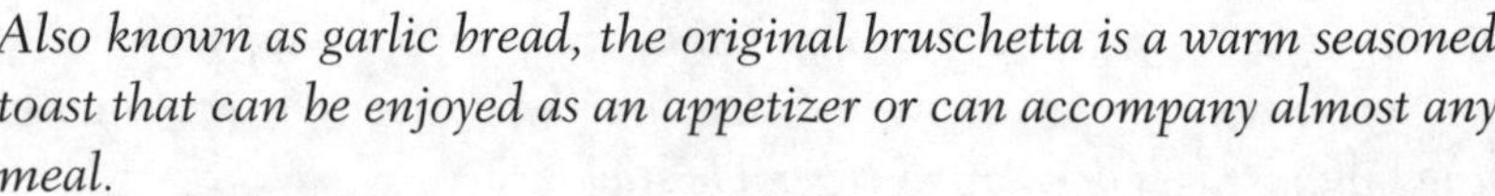

Also known as garlic bread, the original bruschetta is a warm seasoned toast that can be enjoyed as an appetizer or can accompany almost any meal.

1/4 cup extra-virgin olive oil
1/2 teaspoon garlic powder
1 tablespoon chopped fresh parsley
1/2 teaspoon dried-leaf oregano
6 slices crusty Italian or French bread
Salt and pepper, to taste

Preheat broiler or toaster oven. In a small bowl, thoroughly combine oil, garlic powder, parsley, and oregano until well blended. Place bread slices on ungreased baking sheet. Toast bread lightly on both sides. Brush one side of bread with mixture. Place under broiler and brown. Season with salt and pepper. Serve at once. Makes 6 servings.

Each serving contains:

Cal	Prot	Carb	Fib	Tot. Fat	Sat. Fat	Chol	Sodium
136	2g	11g	1g	10g	1g	0mg	166mg

Note: For a stronger garlic flavor, omit garlic powder and rub raw cut garlic cloves over toast before brushing with oil mixture.

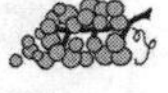

ANCHOVY BRUSCHETTA

Heap this mixture over toast and serve as an appetizer or for lunch along with a mixed green salad.

1 (2-oz.) can anchovies, drained, rinsed
2 teaspoons capers, drained
3 plum (Roma) tomatoes, seeded, chopped
1 tablespoon chopped onion
1 tablespoon chopped fresh parsley
1/4 cup grated Romano cheese
6 slices crusty Italian or French bread

Preheat broiler or toaster oven. Pat drained anchovy fillets with paper towels to dry; chop coarsely. In a bowl, combine all ingredients, except bread. Place bread slices on baking sheet. Toast bread lightly on both sides. Spoon mixture on top and serve at once. Makes 6 servings.

Each serving contains:

Cal	Prot	Carb	Fib	Tot. Fat	Sat. Fat	Chol	Sodium
99	6g	12g	1g	3g	1g	12mg	545mg

Tuna-Stuffed Tomatoes

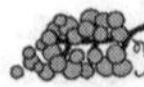 *Start your next party with a colorful tray of stuffed cherry tomatoes.*

1 (7-oz.) can oil-pack tuna, drained
1 green onion, chopped
1 tablespoon chopped cornichons (pickled tiny gherkin cucumbers)
1/4 cup reduced-calorie mayonnaise
1 tablespoon white wine vinegar or pickle vinegar
24 large cherry tomatoes
Chopped fresh parsley

In a small bowl, combine tuna, green onion, cornichons, mayonnaise, and vinegar. Cover and refrigerate. With a sharp knife remove tops of tomatoes. Scoop out seeds and turn tomatoes upside down on paper towels to drain. Fill each tomato with tuna mixture and place on a serving platter. Garnish tops with parsley. Makes 6 four-tomato servings.

Each serving contains:

Cal	Prot	Carb	Fib	Tot. Fat	Sat. Fat	Chol	Sodium
101	9g	5g	1g	5g	1g	13mg	209mg

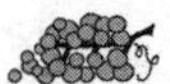

Caponata

A traditional Italian dish, caponata combines a variety of fresh vegetables. I prefer to chill this appetizer overnight, so the flavors can develop more fully.

- 3 tablespoons olive oil
- 1 onion, chopped
- 2 garlic cloves, minced
- 1 (1-lb.) small eggplant, peeled, chopped
- 1 celery stalk, sliced
- 1/4 cup dry-pack sun-dried tomatoes, chopped
- 1 green or yellow bell pepper, chopped
- 2 tomatoes, seeded, chopped
- 1 tablespoon capers, drained
- 1/4 cup red wine vinegar
- 1/4 cup unsalted tomato juice
- 1 tablespoon chopped fresh basil or parsley
- Salt and pepper, to taste

Heat oil in a 12-inch skillet over medium heat. Add onion and garlic and sauté 2 or 3 minutes. Stir in eggplant and celery; sauté, stirring occasionally, until browned. Add remaining ingredients. Reduce heat, cover, and simmer until vegetables are tender, about 20 minutes, stirring occasionally. Serve warm or refrigerate until needed. Caponata may be stored in the refrigerator up to 2 weeks. Makes 6 to 8 servings (about 3 cups).

Each serving contains:

Cal	Prot	Carb	Fib	Tot. Fat	Sat. Fat	Chol	Sodium
114	2g	12g	4g	7g	1g	0mg	153mg

Broccoli Flowers

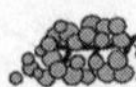

Enjoy this crunchy finger food at your next buffet or picnic.

1 lb. fresh broccoli
2 tablespoons grated Romano cheese
1 tablespoon reduced-calorie mayonnaise
1 tablespoon plain fat-free yogurt
1/2 teaspoon Dijon mustard
1 (5-oz.) package very thinly sliced cooked chicken (about 20 slices)

Trim broccoli; cut flowers and stems into about 20 (3- to 4-inch-long) pieces. Cook in boiling water in a 2-quart saucepan until tender, about 5 minutes; drain. While hot sprinkle with cheese. In a small bowl, combine mayonnaise, yogurt, and mustard. Spread one side of chicken slices with mayonnaise mixture. Place one length of cooked broccoli in center of each chicken slice. Roll up like a cornucopia with broccoli flower protruding through the open end. Serve warm or cold. Makes 6 servings.

Each serving contains:

Cal	Prot	Carb	Fib	Tot. Fat	Sat. Fat	Chol	Sodium
58	7g	5g	1g	1g	0g	11mg	272mg

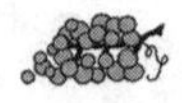

Olive-Stuffed Meatballs

If you choose, make half with almond-stuffed olives and half with pimiento-stuffed olives.

1/2 lb. extra-lean ground beef
1/2 cup cooked bulgur
1 green onion, chopped
1 egg white
1/2 teaspoon dried-leaf basil
1/2 teaspoon dried-leaf marjoram
1 tablespoon chopped parsley
1 tablespoon tomato sauce
20 almond-stuffed olives

In a small mixing bowl, combine beef, bulgur, green onion, egg white, basil, marjoram, parsley, and tomato sauce. Thoroughly mix ingredients. Take a scant tablespoon of meat mixture and pat into a patty; press one olive in center. Pinch meat around olive. Repeat with remaining meat mixture and olives. Warm a 12-inch nonstick sauté pan over medium heat. Cook until browned on all sides. Cover and cook until the interior is no longer pink, 5 minutes. Makes 20 meatballs.

Each meatball contains:

Cal	Prot	Carb	Fib	Tot. Fat	Sat. Fat	Chol	Sodium
36	3g	1g	0g	2g	1g	4mg	124mg

Shrimp-and-Cheese-Stuffed Eggplant Rolls

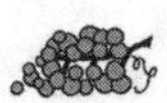

A cool, colorful beginning to that special meal.

1 (1-lb.) eggplant
1/3 cup crumbled herbed feta cheese
1/3 cup ricotta cheese
1 (6-oz.) can cocktail shrimp, drained
1 green onion, chopped
1 tablespoon fresh lemon juice
3 roasted red bell peppers (4 oz.), cut in lengthwise strips
Salt and pepper, to taste
Lettuce leaves
6 teaspoons plain fat-free yogurt
3 teaspoons chopped fresh parsley

Preheat broiler. Lightly spray a baking sheet with olive-oil cooking spray or brush sheet with olive oil. Cut ends off unpeeled eggplant and cut lengthwise into 6 slices. Place slices on baking sheet. Spray lightly. Broil until golden; turn and broil underside. Remove and place on paper towels.

In a bowl, combine the cheeses, shrimp, onion, and lemon juice.

Place red bell pepper strips in a single layer on large ends of eggplant slices. Season with salt and pepper. Spoon shrimp mixture on narrow end of each slice. Carefully roll up, starting at narrow end. Line 6 plates with lettuce leaves. Place an eggplant roll, seam side down, on each lettuce-lined plate and slice in half, exposing spiral filling. If necessary, secure with a wooden pick. To serve, garnish each serving with 1 teaspoon of yogurt and 1/2 teaspoon parsley. Makes 6 servings.

Each serving contains:

Cal	Prot	Carb	Fib	Tot. Fat	Sat. Fat	Chol	Sodium
110	10g	3g	1g	7g	3g	64mg	273mg

As a substitute for prepackaged herbed feta, mix 1/4 teaspoon each of marjoram, basil, and oregano into 1/3 cup of feta cheese.

*M*USHROOM FRITTATA

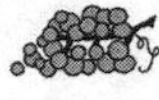

To serve the frittata as an entrée, cut it into larger wedges and top with Caponata, page 57.

- 3 tablespoons olive oil or butter
- 4 green onions, sliced
- 1 garlic clove, minced
- 12 oz. fresh mushrooms, sliced (3 cups)
- 2 eggs, beaten
- 1 tablespoon chopped fresh sage leaves or 1 teaspoon dried
- 1/4 cup Yogurt Cream Cheese, page 62
- 2 tablespoons all-purpose flour
- Salt and pepper, to taste
- 1/4 cup crumbled Gorgonzola or other blue cheese
- Fresh sage leaves, for garnish

Preheat broiler. In a skillet with a flameproof handle, heat oil or butter over medium heat. Add green onions, garlic, and mushrooms and sauté, stirring occasionally, about 5 minutes. Cover and set aside. In a bowl, beat together eggs, chopped sage, Yogurt Cream Cheese, and flour. Season with salt and pepper. Carefully pour egg mixture over mushrooms in skillet.

Return to heat. Cover and cook, without stirring, over medium heat until edges begin to brown. Uncover; sprinkle top with cheese. Place skillet under broiler until cheese melts, 3 to 4 minutes. Serve from skillet or slide frittata onto a warm serving platter. Cut into wedges and garnish with sage leaves. Makes 8 servings.

Each serving contains:

Cal	Prot	Carb	Fib	Tot. Fat	Sat. Fat	Chol	Sodium
101	4g	5g	1g	8g	2g	56mg	108mg

Yogurt Cream Cheese

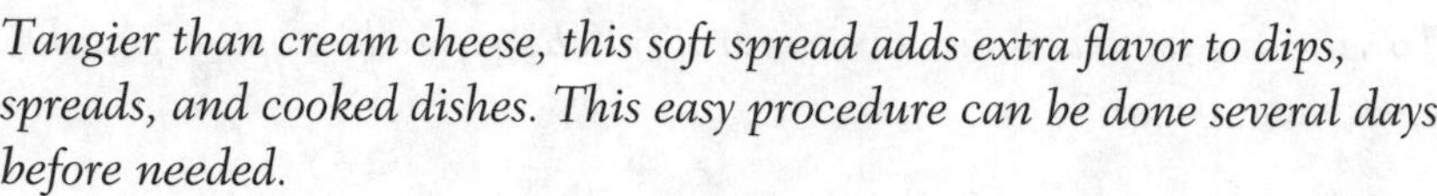

Tangier than cream cheese, this soft spread adds extra flavor to dips, spreads, and cooked dishes. This easy procedure can be done several days before needed.

Caution: Read the yogurt container label. Use only plain yogurt that has not had gelatin or other ingredients added to prohibit the separation of liquid from solids.

2 cups plain fat-free yogurt

Line a sieve or colander with 3 layers of cheesecloth or paper coffee filters. Place sieve over a bowl. Add yogurt and cover. Let drain, refrigerated, for 4 to 6 hours. Discard liquid. Store yogurt in a container with a lid. This can be stored in the refrigerator for up to 10 days. Makes 1 cup.

Each tablespoon contains:

Cal	Prot	Carb	Fib	Tot. Fat	Sat. Fat	Chol	Sodium
12	1g	2g	0g	0g	0g	1mg	17mg

Walnut-Topped Portobello Mushrooms

Portobellos, robust meaty mushrooms, can serve as a meat substitute.

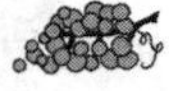

8 oz. (4) Portobello mushrooms
2 anchovy fillets (1 oz.), rinsed
1 tablespoon balsamic vinegar
3 tablespoons olive oil
1 garlic clove, minced
2 tablespoons chopped walnuts

Brush mushrooms with a paper towel to clean. Remove stems and set mushrooms in a shallow flameproof baking dish. Pat anchovy fillets to remove excess moisture. In a cup, combine vinegar, olive oil, and garlic. Add anchovies and mash into mixture. Brush both sides of mushrooms with anchovy mixture; let stand at least 15 minutes. Turn in marinade several times.

Preheat broiler or grill. Broil mushrooms, top side up, for 5 minutes. Turn and brush gill side with marinade and sprinkle with walnuts. Broil another 3 to 4 minutes. Serve at once. Makes 4 servings.

Each serving contains:

Cal	Prot	Carb	Fib	Tot. Fat	Sat. Fat	Chol	Sodium
145	5g	4g	2g	13g	2g	6mg	268mg

Hummus

The bean in this recipe has three names: It's known as chickpea, ceci bean, or garbanzo bean. This nutritious bean is a mainstay in Middle Eastern, Indian, and Mediterranean cuisines. Use this recipe as a dip or spread.

1 (15-oz.) can garbanzo beans, drained
1/4 cup fresh lemon juice
1/2 teaspoon garlic powder or 2 garlic cloves, minced
1 tablespoon chopped fresh parsley
1/2 teaspoon dried-leaf marjoram or basil
1/4 teaspoon sugar (optional)
1/4 teaspoon dried red chile pepper flakes (optional)
1 tablespoon olive oil (optional)
Salt and pepper, to taste

In a blender or food processor, combine all ingredients. Pulse or blend to desired consistency, adding a little water if necessary. Scrape down the sides of the container as necessary. Makes 8 servings (about 1-1/2 cups).

Each serving contains:

Cal	Prot	Carb	Fib	Tot. Fat	Sat. Fat	Chol	Sodium
51	3g	9g	2g	1g	0g	0mg	161mg

Soups

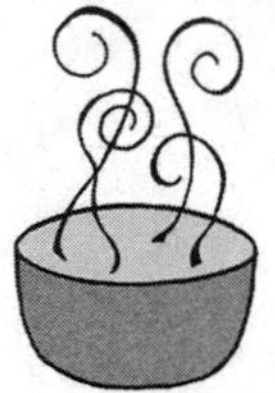

Cool weather seems to call for homemade soup. For many of us, it brings back memories of home and tasty, nourishing simple meals. Somehow canned soups can't compare to your own home-cooked ones. Artichoke-Hazelnut Soup offers a different combination of flavors. For something out of the ordinary, serve French Eggplant and Bean Soup; it uses the everyday ingredients found in the Provence region of France.

The popular cold soups are probably enjoyed most during warm weather. One that is especially refreshing is the delicately colored Cucumber Gazpacho. This can be prepared ahead and refrigerated until needed. However, if you choose to showcase this at your next outdoor gathering, give it a special presentation. Fill a large bowl with ice and nestle your serving bowl or tureen in the center. Tuck fresh greens into the ice surrounding the bowl. Place condiments around the bowl and let everyone garnish their own portion.

An example of a meal in a bowl is the wonderful Cioppino, an Italian seafood soup. It's fun to let guests try to identify all the different ingredients. For hearty soups, I suggest Lentil and Broccoli Soup or Country Vegetable Soup. For a simply satisfying lunch, pour soup into large cups and serve with thick slices of warm French bread and follow with a mixed green salad. Let the recipe for Fresh Mushroom Soup be the basis for any creamed vegetable soup. It's a

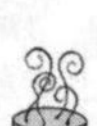

great way to transform small amounts of leftovers into a delicious cream soup. A way to extend soup is to add beans, rice, or pasta, thus making a complete meal.

Always bear in mind that recipes are merely your guides. Feel free to make substitutions, creating your own original dish.

Artichoke-Hazelnut Soup

Cooks throughout the Mediterranean use artichokes. Enjoy this combination of subtle flavors.

1 tablespoon olive oil
1/2 cup chopped onion
1 garlic clove, crushed
1 (8-oz.) can artichokes, chopped, drained or 1 (10-oz.) package frozen, thawed
2 cups reduced-sodium canned chicken broth
1/2 teaspoon dried-leaf oregano
1/2 cup roasted, chopped hazelnuts
3 tablespoons all-purpose flour
1-1/2 cups evaporated fat-free milk
1/2 cup vermouth or white wine
Salt and pepper, to taste
2 tablespoons crumbled herbed feta cheese

In a 3-quart nonstick saucepan, heat oil over medium heat. Add onion and garlic and sauté until softened. Add artichokes, broth, oregano, and hazelnuts. Cook until tender, about 5 minutes. Blend flour in evaporated milk and vermouth or white wine; add to mixture and cook, stirring, until slightly thickened, 5 to 7 minutes. Season with salt and pepper. Garnish with feta cheese. Serve hot. Makes 5 (1-cup) servings.

Each serving contains:

Cal	Prot	Carb	Fib	Tot. Fat	Sat. Fat	Chol	Sodium
255	12g	22g	4g	12g	2g	6mg	533mg

Fresh Mushroom Soup

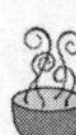

For a more interesting taste and appearance, alter this recipe by using three different kinds of mushrooms.

3 tablespoons butter
1/4 onion, chopped
1 garlic clove, minced
3/4 lb. fresh mushrooms, sliced
4 cups reduced-sodium chicken broth
1/2 teaspoon dried-leaf thyme
1/3 cup all-purpose flour
1-1/2 cups fat-free milk
1/4 cup white wine
Salt and pepper, to taste
1/4 cup grated Parmesan cheese

In a 3-quart nonstick saucepan, melt butter or margarine over medium heat. Add onion, garlic, and mushrooms and sauté, stirring occasionally, until mushrooms are lightly browned. Add broth and thyme. Reduce heat and simmer about 20 minutes. Remove pan from heat. Blend flour and milk. Stir flour mixture and wine into broth mixture. Simmer, stirring, until slightly thickened, 5 to 7 minutes. Season with salt and pepper. Stir in Parmesan cheese. Serve hot. Makes 6 (1-cup) servings.

Each serving contains:

Cal	Prot	Carb	Fib	Tot. Fat	Sat. Fat	Chol	Sodium
175	9g	12g	1g	9g	5g	24mg	678mg

Spinach, Zucchini, and Bean Soup

This soup is especially good with toasted slices of French, Italian, or pita bread.

2 teaspoons olive oil
1/2 cup diced onion
3 carrots, sliced
2 cups sliced zucchini
4 cups water or reduced-sodium canned beef broth
1 bay leaf
2 fresh tomatoes, chopped
1 (15-oz.) can pink kidney or pinto beans, drained
1 bunch fresh spinach, stems removed, chopped or 1 (10-oz.) package chopped frozen, thawed, and drained
2 tablespoons chopped fresh parsley
1/2 cup cooked small pasta shells
Salt, to taste

Heat oil in a large saucepan or stockpot over medium heat. Add onion, carrots, and zucchini; sauté, stirring occasionally, until softened. Add water or broth and bay leaf. Bring mixture to full boil, partially cover, reduce heat, and simmer 20 minutes. Add tomatoes and beans and cook until vegetables are tender, about 10 minutes. Remove from heat, add spinach, parsley, and pasta; cover and let stand 10 minutes. Remove and discard bay leaf. Season with salt. Serve hot. Makes 8 (1-cup) servings.

Each serving contains:

Cal	Prot	Carb	Fib	Tot. Fat	Sat. Fat	Chol	Sodium
127	6g	22g	8g	2g	0g	0mg	88mg

Country Vegetable Soup

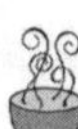

Serve a warm and satisfying meal in a bowl—it's ideal for a cold day.

1 tablespoon olive oil
1 onion, chopped
2 celery stalks, chopped
2 carrots, sliced
1/2 cup canned garbanzo beans (chickpeas)
1 (8-oz.) can tomatoes with juice
2 bay leaves
1/2 teaspoon Italian herbs
2 cups reduced-sodium canned chicken broth
1 cup unsalted tomato juice
5 cups water
1 tablespoon fresh chopped parsley
1/2 cup fresh sliced mushrooms

In a 5-1/2-quart nonstick Dutch oven, heat oil. Sauté onion, celery, and carrots until softened. Add beans, tomatoes with juice, bay leaves, Italian herbs, broth, tomato juice, and water. Bring to a boil, reduce heat, and cook over medium heat until vegetables are tender, about 30 minutes. Add parsley and mushrooms. Cook another 7 to 10 minutes. Remove and discard bay leaves. Serve hot. Makes 8 (1-cup) servings.

Each serving contains:

Cal	Prot	Carb	Fib	Tot. Fat	Sat. Fat	Chol	Sodium
66	3g	9g	2g	3g	0g	0mg	259mg

Chestnut Soup

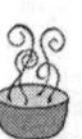

Chestnuts are a frequent ingredient in Italian desserts and savory dishes.

2 teaspoons olive or canola oil
1/2 onion, chopped
1 carrot, sliced
1 celery stalk, sliced
4 cups reduced-sodium canned chicken broth or homemade turkey broth
1 teaspoon sugar
1 bay leaf
1/4 teaspoon dried-leaf basil
1/8 teaspoon dried-leaf marjoram
24 (about 1/2 lb. total) fresh chestnuts, roasted, shelled (see "Chestnuts" box, page 72)
1/2 cup evaporated fat-free milk
3/4 cup marsala, sherry, or water
Salt and pepper, to taste

In a 5-1/2-quart nonstick Dutch oven, heat oil over medium heat. Add onion, carrot, and celery and sauté until softened. Add broth, sugar, bay leaf, basil, marjoram, and chestnuts. Simmer until chestnuts are tender, about 25 minutes. Remove and discard bay leaf. Carefully transfer mixture to a food processor or blender and purée. Return to pot, stir in evaporated milk, and bring to a boil. Add marsala, sherry, or water. Season with salt and pepper. Serve hot or cold. Makes 6 (1-cup) servings.

Each serving contains:

Cal	Prot	Carb	Fib	Tot. Fat	Sat. Fat	Chol	Sodium
206	6g	30g	3g	3g	1g	1mg	604mg

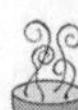

Chestnuts

Whole chestnuts are available fresh, canned, and dried. To roast fresh chestnuts: Preheat oven to 425˚F (220˚C). Cut an X in the flat side of each chestnut with the tip of a knife (this will prevent the chestnut from exploding when the liquid in the chestnut turns to steam as it is heated). Place in a baking pan. Roast about 20 minutes or until chestnuts are tender, stirring once or twice. Cool slightly and peel off the dark outer shell and papery skin. Fresh chestnuts are usually available from about October to February; they are perishable and must be stored in a cool area. If you are fortunate enough to have your own chestnut tree or have a friend with one, fresh chestnuts can be boiled or baked, then cooled and frozen in freezer containers. Canned chestnuts and rehydrated dried chestnuts can be substituted for fresh ones.

Chestnuts are also available as chestnut flour and chestnut purée, both sweetened and unsweetened.

Cioppino

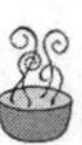

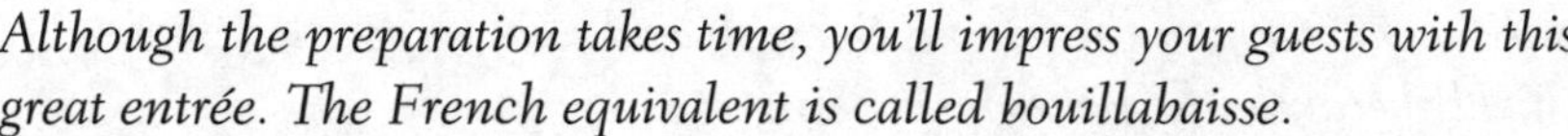

Although the preparation takes time, you'll impress your guests with this great entrée. The French equivalent is called bouillabaisse.

1 tablespoon olive oil
1/2 cup chopped celery
1 onion, chopped
2 garlic cloves, crushed
1/2 cup chopped fresh parsley
2 (8-oz.) cans low-sodium tomato sauce
2 cups water
3 large fresh tomatoes, chopped
1/2 teaspoon dried-leaf basil
1/4 teaspoon dried-leaf marjoram
3/4 cup red wine or tomato juice
4 fresh or frozen crab legs, cut into halves
1 lb. fresh clams, scrubbed
1 lb. peeled shrimp
1 lb. rock cod, cut into 1-inch cubes
Salt and pepper to taste

In a 5-1/2-quart nonstick Dutch oven, heat oil over medium heat. Add celery, onion, and garlic and sauté until softened. Add parsley, tomato sauce, water, tomatoes, basil, marjoram, and wine or tomato juice. Simmer until vegetables are tender, 20 to 25 minutes. Add crab, clams, and shrimp; cook 5 minutes. Add cod and cook until tender but not falling apart, 5 to 7 minutes. Season with salt and pepper, adding more wine if desired. Discard any clams that do not open. Serve hot. Makes 8 (1-cup) servings.

Each serving contains:

Cal	Prot	Carb	Fib	Tot. Fat	Sat. Fat	Chol	Sodium
306	46g	13g	2g	5g	1g	166mg	925mg

Cucumber Gazpacho

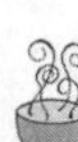

A white variation of the famous Spanish cold soup; it goes together quickly because it requires no cooking.

1 garlic clove, peeled
2 large cucumbers, peeled, seeded, sliced
2 cups reduced-sodium canned chicken broth
1 cup plain fat-free yogurt
1 cup fat-free dairy sour cream
2 tablespoons white vinegar
Salt and pepper, to taste
2 tablespoons chopped pimiento
2 green onions, chopped
1/4 cup sliced almonds, toasted or raw

In a food processor or blender, combine garlic, cucumbers, and 1/4 cup of the broth; purée. Add remaining broth, yogurt, sour cream, and vinegar. Pour into a serving bowl and season with salt and pepper. Serve at once or cover and chill until needed or for up to 24 hours. Spoon into individual bowls and garnish with pimiento, green onions, and almonds. Makes 6 to 8 servings.

Each serving contains:

Cal	Prot	Carb	Fib	Tot. Fat	Sat. Fat	Chol	Sodium
110	7g	14g	1g	3g	0g	1mg	363mg

Lentil and Broccoli Soup

Extra spices give zest to this hearty dish. Lentils are a good source of fiber and protein.

1 cup dried lentils
1/2 onion, chopped
1/2 teaspoon cardamom
1 carrot, sliced
1 celery stalk, sliced
1/2 teaspoon black pepper
1 red bell pepper, sliced
1/2 teaspoon ground cinnamon
4 cups canned vegetable broth
4 cups water
4 tomatoes, seeded, chopped
1 (10-oz.) package frozen chopped broccoli

Rinse and sort lentils. In a 5-1/2-quart nonstick Dutch oven, combine lentils, onion, cardamom, carrot, celery, black pepper, bell pepper, cinnamon, broth, and water. Bring to a boil. Cover, reduce heat, and simmer until lentils are done, about 30 minutes. Add tomatoes and broccoli and simmer until tender, about 10 minutes. Season with salt. Serve hot. Makes 8 (1-cup) servings.

Each serving contains:

Cal	Prot	Carb	Fib	Tot. Fat	Sat. Fat	Chol	Sodium
113	8g	21g	7g	1g	0g	0g	1,692mg

Note: If you use homemade vegetable broth, then sodium will decrease significantly.

French Eggplant and Bean Soup

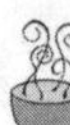

Most of the eggplants grown in France and Italy are the smaller varieties.

1 small eggplant
4 tablespoons olive oil
1/2 onion, chopped
1 red bell pepper, chopped
8 cups (2 quarts) reduced-sodium canned chicken broth
1 bay leaf
1/2 teaspoon dried-leaf oregano
2 large tomatoes, chopped
1 (10-oz.) package frozen baby lima beans
Grated Parmesan cheese, for garnish

Peel eggplant and cut into 1/2-inch cubes. Heat olive oil in a 3-quart nonstick saucepan over medium heat. Add eggplant and brown, turning. Add onion, bell pepper, broth, bay leaf, oregano, tomatoes, and beans. Bring to a full boil. Reduce heat, cover, and simmer until eggplant is very soft, about 15 minutes. Remove bay leaf before serving. If desired, pour half of mixture into a food processor and purée and return to pot. Serve hot with Parmesan cheese. Makes 5 (1-cup) servings.

Each serving contains:

Cal	Prot	Carb	Fib	Tot. Fat	Sat. Fat	Chol	Sodium
225	12g	18g	5g	12g	2g	2mg	1,095mg

Note: If you use homemade chicken broth, then sodium will decrease significantly.

Beef, Barley, and Tomato Soup

Fresh fennel adds distinction to a traditional soup.

1 lb. boneless short ribs or beef shank, cubed
6 cups reduced-sodium canned beef broth or 3 cups broth and 3 cups water
2 cups water
1 onion, chopped
1 fennel, trimmed, sliced
2 celery stalks, chopped
1/4 cup sun-dried tomatoes, chopped
1 (14-1/4-oz.) can tomatoes, chopped
1/2 cup pearl barley
1/2 teaspoon dried-leaf oregano
Salt and pepper, to taste
1/2 cup cooked kidney beans
2 tablespoons chopped fresh parsley

Brown beef cubes in a 5-quart nonstick Dutch oven or stockpot over medium heat. Add 2 cups of the broth, cover, and cook 15 minutes. Add remaining ingredients, except kidney beans and parsley. Cover and simmer until meat and vegetables are tender, about 1 hour. Add beans and parsley; cook 5 minutes. Serve hot. Makes 8 (1-cup) servings.

Each serving contains:

Cal	Prot	Carb	Fib	Tot. Fat	Sat. Fat	Chol	Sodium
368	18g	19g	5g	24g	10g	53mg	752mg

Note: If you use homemade beef broth, then sodium will decrease significantly.

Chicken and Rice Soup

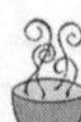

Mothers around the world serve their own version of chicken soup—this one is very simple but packed with flavor.

2 teaspoons olive oil
3 green onions, chopped
1 celery stalk, sliced
1 carrot, shredded
1/2 cup long-grain white rice
4 cups reduced-sodium canned chicken broth
2 cups water
1 cup cooked, shredded chicken
1 tablespoon chopped fresh basil or parsley
Salt and pepper, to taste
Cooked fine egg noodles (optional)

Heat oil in a 3-quart saucepan over medium heat. Add onions, celery, and carrot and sauté until softened. Add rice, broth, water, and chicken. Simmer uncovered until rice is tender, about 15 minutes. Stir in basil or parsley and season with salt and pepper. Ladle hot soup into bowls and add noodles, if desired. Makes 8 (1-cup) servings.

Each serving contains:

Cal	Prot	Carb	Fib	Tot. Fat	Sat. Fat	Chol	Sodium
112	9g	11g	1g	4g	1g	20mg	410mg

Creamed Asparagus–Rice Soup

If you'd like it a bit spicier, add 1/2 teaspoon dried red chile flakes.

1 tablespoon olive oil
1/2 onion, chopped
1 lb. fresh asparagus, trimmed or 1 (10-oz.) package frozen
1/2 cup cooked chicken, chopped
1/4 red bell pepper, chopped
4 cups reduced-sodium canned chicken broth
2 cups water
1/4 cup long-grain white rice
1/4 teaspoon grated nutmeg
1-1/2 cups evaporated fat-free milk
3 tablespoons all-purpose flour
Salt and pepper, to taste

Heat oil in a nonstick 5-quart Dutch oven or stockpot over medium heat. Add onion and sauté until softened. Add asparagus, chicken, bell pepper, broth, water, rice, and nutmeg. Cover and reduce heat. Simmer until rice and vegetables are tender, 20 to 25 minutes. In a small bowl, blend milk and flour. Stir into soup mixture, and simmer, stirring, until lightly thickened. Season with salt and pepper. Serve hot. Makes 6 to 8 servings.

Each serving contains:

Cal	Prot	Carb	Fib	Tot. Fat	Sat. Fat	Chol	Sodium
184	14g	22g	2g	5g	1g	12mg	652mg

Salads

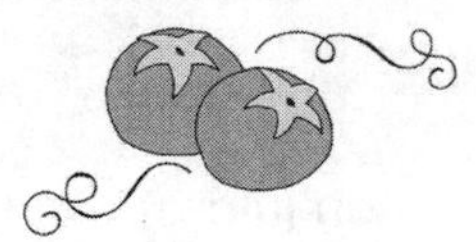

Even a plain mixed green salad becomes a real treat when served fresh, crisp, and chilled, topped lightly with a delicious dressing. Salads can be served as an appetizer, main dish, or side dish or as a palate cleanser after the entrée.

What a wonderful way to enrich your daily diet! Your salad can become a meal in itself when it contains protein. This is easily accomplished by adding cheese, meat, beans, or eggs. Examples are the Greek Salad and Chicken, Melon, and Grape Salad.

Do try some of the wonderful greens that are now available. They may not be familiar to you, but they have long been standards in Mediterranean kitchens. They offer subtle differences in flavor, as well as vibrant colors. For more robust flavor, choose Romaine or peppery chicory (curly endive). For added interest, include contrasting colors; for example, red leaf lettuce or the beautiful deep-red radicchio (Italian chicory) with its white veins. In general, these eye-catching ingredients are more expensive, but they can be used in combination with less expensive greens.

Frugal housewives use day-old bread as the main ingredient in Panzanella (bread salad), which can be varied depending on the types of fresh vegetables available that day.

Delight everyone at the table by garnishing your salad now and then with edible flowers such as nasturtium, borage, or pot marigold.

ASPARAGUS, ALMOND, AND RAISIN SALAD

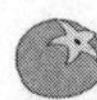

The subtle flavor of chilled asparagus is accented, but not overpowered, by raisins and almonds.

1 bunch fresh spinach or salad mixed greens
1 lb. cooked asparagus
1 tomato, chopped
1 tablespoon fresh lemon juice
1 tablespoon chopped fresh parsley
1 tablespoon slivered blanched almonds
1 tablespoon dark raisins
1/3 cup Balsamic Herb Dressing, page 103

Rinse spinach or salad greens and pat dry. Line salad plates with spinach or greens. Combine asparagus with tomato, lemon juice, and parsley. Divide evenly over spinach, then sprinkle with almonds and raisins. Drizzle with Balsamic Herb Dressing. Makes 6 side servings.

Each serving contains:

Cal	Prot	Carb	Fib	Tot. Fat	Sat. Fat	Chol	Sodium
112	4g	9g	3g	8g	1g	0mg	57mg

Cucumber, Tomato, and Onion Salad

For a special treat, add thick orange slices to this simple salad. Serve it in a glass bowl so the vibrant colors will be noticed.

2 tablespoons olive oil
1/3 cup cider vinegar
5 tablespoons water
5 tablespoons sugar
2 large cucumbers, thinly sliced
2 large tomatoes, sliced
1 red onion, thinly sliced
Salt and pepper, to taste
Fresh dill, for garnish

Combine all ingredients in a large glass bowl. Cover and refrigerate at least 1 hour or up to 6 hours before serving. Makes 6 side servings.

Each serving contains:

Cal	Prot	Carb	Fib	Tot. Fat	Sat. Fat	Chol	Sodium
113	1g	18g	2g	5g	1g	0mg	57mg

Warm Garbanzo and Pasta Salad

I like to serve this salad warm, but it's equally delicious chilled.

2 tablespoons olive oil
2 green onions, chopped
1/2 cup green bell pepper, sliced
2 tablespoons oil-pack sun-dried tomatoes, chopped
1/2 teaspoon dried-leaf oregano
1 (15-oz.) can garbanzo beans (chickpeas), drained, rinsed
1/4 cup fresh lemon juice
1–1/2 cups warm cooked pasta
2 tablespoons chopped fresh parsley
10 small black olives, sliced
1 tomato, seeded, chopped

Heat oil in an 8-inch nonstick fry pan over medium heat. Add green onions and bell pepper and sauté until softened. Stir in sun-dried tomatoes, oregano, and garbanzo beans and remove from heat. In a large bowl, toss together bean mixture, lemon juice, pasta, parsley, and olives. Stir and sprinkle top with tomato. Serve warm or chilled. Makes 8 (1/2-cup) servings.

Each serving contains:

Cal	Prot	Carb	Fib	Tot. Fat	Sat. Fat	Chol	Sodium
142	4g	21g	3g	5g	1g	0mg	194mg

SALAD NIÇOISE

My version of the French classic salad is tossed together for easy assembly and serving.

2 cups cut green beans, crisp cooked
1 cup sliced fresh mushrooms (about 1/2 lb.)
2 cups sliced, peeled, cooked potatoes
3 green onions, chopped
2 tablespoons capers, drained
12 black olives
1 (6-oz.) can oil-packed tuna, drained
2 tomatoes, sliced
1 (2-oz.) can anchovies, drained, chopped
1/3 cup Red Wine Vinaigrette dressing, page 106

In a large salad bowl, toss all ingredients. Cover and refrigerate at least 2 hours before serving. Makes 6 (1-cup) servings.

Each serving contains:

Cal	Prot	Carb	Fib	Tot. Fat	Sat. Fat	Chol	Sodium
222	13g	17g	3g	12g	2g	16mg	585mg

Shrimp and White Bean Salad

White beans and seafood make a classic combination for a main-dish salad. The beans add fiber and additional protein.

1 (16-oz.) can cannellini (white kidney) beans or 1 cup cooked small white beans, drained
1 (6-oz.) can cocktail shrimp or water-pack tuna, drained
1 cup sliced green bell pepper
1/2 red onion, chopped
2 celery stalks, sliced
1 large tomato, chopped
1 tablespoon chopped green olives
1/2 cup Italian Dressing, page 107
Shredded red cabbage

Rinse drained beans with water and drain again. In a salad bowl, stir all ingredients together, except cabbage. Cover and chill. Line 8 salad plates with cabbage and spoon bean and shrimp mixture on top. Makes 8 servings.

Each serving contains:

Cal	Prot	Carb	Fib	Tot. Fat	Sat. Fat	Chol	Sodium
149	8g	12g	3g	8g	1g	37mg	192mg

FRUIT AND CABBAGE SALAD

A crisp cabbage salad provides a welcome contrast of textures when paired with soft or creamed dishes.

1-1/2 cups shredded red cabbage
1-1/2 cups shredded green cabbage
2 green onions, sliced
1 apple, cored, sliced
1/2 cup Zante currants
1/2 cup green grapes
2 celery stalks, sliced
1 teaspoon fennel seeds
2/3 cup Balsamic Herb Dressing, page 103

In a salad bowl, mix red and green cabbage, green onions, apple, currants, grapes, celery, and fennel seeds. Pour Balsamic Herb Dressing over and toss to coat. Makes 6 side servings.

Each serving contains:

Cal	Prot	Carb	Fib	Tot. Fat	Sat. Fat	Chol	Sodium
199	2g	20g	3g	14g	2g	0mg	22mg

Couscous Fruit Salad

This North African pasta cousin is precooked, granular semolina. Here it's combined with fruit and spices—a nice way to introduce couscous to those who haven't enjoyed it before.

1-1/4 cups orange juice
1/4 teaspoon ground cinnamon
1/4 teaspoon freshly grated nutmeg
1 cup dry couscous
1/4 cup dark raisins
1 cup chopped dried apricots
1 cup seedless red grapes
1 orange, peeled, segmented
1/2 avocado, chopped
2 teaspoons fresh lemon juice
3 tablespoons toasted slivered almonds

Place orange juice, cinnamon, and nutmeg in a 1-quart nonstick saucepan; bring to a boil. Stir in couscous, raisins, and apricots. Cover and remove from heat. Let stand 5 minutes. Spoon mixture into a serving bowl. Top with grapes. Garnish with orange segments and avocado. Sprinkle lemon juice and almonds on top. Makes 6 side servings.

Each serving contains:

Cal	Prot	Carb	Fib	Tot. Fat	Sat. Fat	Chol	Sodium
284	7g	56g	6g	6g	1g	0mg	10mg

MARINATED DATES AND FIGS WITH SPINACH AND FENNEL

Fennel bulbs resemble large flat celery stalks but have a distinctive licorice flavor.

1/3 cup chopped dried white figs
1/3 cup chopped dates
1/2 cup Italian Dressing, page 107
1 bunch fresh spinach
1/4 head red leaf lettuce
1 fennel (sweet anise) bulb, trimmed and sliced
2 tablespoons chopped roasted hazelnuts

Place figs and dates in a small bowl; cover with Italian Dressing. Wash spinach and lettuce and remove stems. Pat leaves dry with paper towels. Tear into pieces. Place spinach, lettuce, and fennel slices in a serving bowl. Drain figs and dates, reserving dressing. Add fruit and hazelnuts to bowl; toss to combinc. If desired, add reserved dressing. Makes 4 side servings.

Each serving contains:

Cal	Prot	Carb	Fib	Tot. Fat	Sat. Fat	Chol	Sodium
270	5g	31g	8g	17g	2g	0mg	102mg

Greek Salad

This healthful salad gets my vote for the ideal summer luncheon dish.

2 cucumbers, sliced
1/2 green bell pepper, sliced
1/2 onion, chopped
3 tomatoes, chopped
4 radishes, sliced
1 tablespoon capers, drained
1/2 teaspoon dried-leaf oregano
2 tablespoons white wine vinegar
4 tablespoons olive oil
1 oz. feta cheese, crumbled
12 black Greek olives

In a large bowl, combine all ingredients. Cover and chill about 1 hour. Serve with crusty French bread. Makes 4 main dish servings.

Each serving contains:

Cal	Prot	Carb	Fib	Tot. Fat	Sat. Fat	Chol	Sodium
208	3g	12g	2g	18g	3g	6mg	290mg

MEDITERRANEAN VEGETABLE SALAD

If you have a garden, chances are you'll have most of these vegetables.

1 large green bell pepper, sliced
1 large zucchini, sliced
1/2 cup sliced mushrooms
6 radishes, sliced
1 tablespoon chopped Italian parsley
12 small pitted green olives
1 tablespoon olive oil
1 tablespoon red wine vinegar
1/2 teaspoon black pepper
Bibb lettuce
1/4 cup grated Parmesan cheese

Combine first four vegetables, parsley, and olives in a bowl. Mix well. Sprinkle vegetables with olive oil, vinegar, and black pepper. Toss well. Cover and chill about 1 hour. Serve on lettuce leaves, topped with Parmesan cheese. Makes 6 side servings.

Each serving contains:

Cal	Prot	Carb	Fib	Tot. Fat	Sat. Fat	Chol	Sodium
66	3g	4g	1g	5g	1g	3mg	269mg

Artichoke, Carrot, and Orange Salad

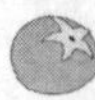

Carrots and orange add a dash of color as well as flavor to this eye-appealing salad.

1/4 cup cider vinegar
1/4 cup olive or canola oil
1/3 cup sugar
1 teaspoon dry mustard
1/2 teaspoon fennel seeds
1 teaspoon grated onion
1/4 teaspoon salt
1 (9-oz.) package frozen artichokes, cooked, drained
1 carrot, shredded
1 medium orange, peeled, cut into rounds

In a 1-quart nonstick saucepan, combine vinegar, oil, sugar, dry mustard, fennel seeds, onion, and salt. Stir over medium heat until sugar dissolves. Cool to room temperature. Combine artichokes, carrot, and orange in large bowl. Pour dressing over; toss to coat. Makes 6 or 7 side servings.

Each serving contains:

Cal	Prot	Carb	Fib	Tot. Fat	Sat. Fat	Chol	Sodium
160	2g	19g	3g	10g	1g	0mg	121mg

TRI-PEPPER POTATO SALAD

Brighten your meal with this great salad.

1/2 cup French Dressing, page 104
3 potatoes, cooked, peeled, cubed (4 cups)
1 red bell pepper, julienned
1 yellow or orange bell pepper, julienned
1 green bell pepper, julienned
2 green onions, chopped
1 cup sliced fresh mushrooms
1 tablespoon chopped fresh basil or 1 teaspoon dried-leaf basil
1/2 cup cooked or canned garbanzo beans, drained
Spinach leaves or Romaine lettuce
1 tablespoon toasted pumpkin seeds

Pour French Dressing over potatoes in a large bowl and marinate at least 1 hour. Add remaining ingredients, except spinach leaves and pumpkin seeds, tossing to combine. Line a salad bowl with spinach or lettuce leaves. Place salad on top of leaves. Sprinkle with pumpkin seeds. Makes 6 side servings.

Each serving contains:

Cal	Prot	Carb	Fib	Tot. Fat	Sat. Fat	Chol	Sodium
223	5g	30g	4g	11g	1g	0mg	107mg

Potato-Artichoke Salad

Substitute cucumber for zucchini, if zucchini is not available.

3 red potatoes, cooked, peeled, cubed (4 cups)
1/2 red onion, chopped
2 tomatoes, thinly sliced
1 (6-1/4-oz.) jar marinated artichokes, drained
2 tablespoons olive oil
2 tablespoons fresh lemon juice
1/4 teaspoon garlic powder
1/4 teaspoon dill weed
1 tablespoon chopped fresh basil or 1 teaspoon dried-leaf basil
1 tablespoon pine nuts

In a salad bowl, combine potatoes, onion, tomatoes, and artichokes. In a cup, blend oil, lemon juice, garlic powder, dill weed, and basil. Pour over potato mixture and toss gently to combine. Sprinkle with pine nuts. Cover and chill before serving. Makes 4 to 6 side servings.

Each serving contains:

Cal	Prot	Carb	Fib	Tot. Fat	Sat. Fat	Chol	Sodium
251	5g	35g	5g	12g	2g	0mg	256mg

Cantaloupe, Summer Berries, and Ricotta Salad

Fresh ripe melons are enhanced with cheese and berries. Try this for a special breakfast.

1 cantaloupe
1 cup reduced-fat ricotta cheese
1/4 cup orange juice
16 blackberries
16 strawberries, halved
1/2 cup Honey–Poppy Seed Dressing, page 105

Peel cantaloupe and cut into 16 lengthwise slices. Divide them equally among 4 plates. In a small bowl, stir cheese and orange juice together. Mound cheese mixture on top of melon slices. Garnish with blackberries and strawberries. Drizzle with Honey–Poppy Seed Dressing. Makes 4 main dish servings.

Each serving without dressing contains:

Cal	Prot	Carb	Fib	Tot. Fat	Sat. Fat	Chol	Sodium
290	9g	43g	4g	11g	3g	19mg	103mg

Pear and Blue Cheese Salad

Grapefruit and pears combine in a splendid winter salad.

Lettuce leaves
2 pears, halved, sliced
1/2 cup Honey–Poppy Seed Dressing, page 105
1/2 cup seedless green grapes
1/2 cup crumbled blue cheese
2 tablespoons pomegranate seeds
2 tablespoons toasted chopped almonds

Arrange lettuce leaves on 4 salad plates. Top with pear slices. Sprinkle dressing over each salad. Top with grapes, cheese, pomegranate seeds, and almonds. Makes 4 side servings.

Each serving contains:

Cal	Prot	Carb	Fib	Tot. Fat	Sat. Fat	Chol	Sodium
275	6g	39g	3g	13g	4g	13mg	240mg

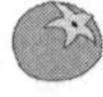

PANZANELLA

Leftover bread plus salad ingredients equals a wonderful entrée. You can also add a small amount of chopped salami or roasted bell peppers.

1 garlic clove, minced
3 tablespoons olive oil
1 tablespoon red wine vinegar
1/4 teaspoon dry mustard
1 tablespoon chopped fresh oregano
2 cups cubed leftover French or Italian bread
1 green onion, chopped
2 large tomatoes, seeded, chopped
4 oz. mozzarella cheese, diced
1/2 cooked or canned pink kidney beans, drained
1 bunch Romaine lettuce, torn
8 black olives, pitted, chopped

In a cup, combine garlic, oil, vinegar, mustard, and oregano. Set aside. In a large bowl, combine all remaining ingredients. Pour dressing over all and toss thoroughly. Let stand at least 10 minutes or up to 30 minutes for bread to absorb dressing. Makes 4 main dish servings.

Each serving contains:

Cal	Prot	Carb	Fib	Tot. Fat	Sat. Fat	Chol	Sodium
321	12g	27g	5g	19g	5g	22mg	343mg

Chicken, Melon, and Grape Salad

A cool, light main-dish salad, it has lots of good-for-you fruits and vegetables. Serve with bread and a cold drink.

1 celery stalk, sliced
1 cucumber, peeled, sliced
1/2 cantaloupe, peeled, cubed
1/2 green bell pepper, chopped
1/2 cup red seedless grapes
1 cup cubed cooked chicken
1/4 head red leaf lettuce, torn in bite-size pieces
1/3 cup French Dressing, page 104

Combine celery, cucumber, cantaloupe, bell pepper, grapes, and chicken in large bowl. Cover and refrigerate until chilled. Add lettuce and dressing and toss to combine. Spoon onto serving plates. Makes 4 main dish servings.

Each serving contains:

Cal	Prot	Carb	Fib	Tot. Fat	Sat. Fat	Chol	Sodium
209	12g	16g	2g	8g	1g	29mg	126mg

SHRIMP AND SCALLOPS WITH CUCUMBERS AND CHERRY TOMATOES

Treat yourself to this chilled seafood salad.

Lettuce or spinach leaves
1/2 cup cooked shrimp
1/2 cup cooked scallops
2 celery stalks, sliced
1 green onion, finely chopped
1 tablespoon chopped fresh parsley
1 tablespoon fresh lemon or lime juice
1 cucumber, sliced
12 cherry tomatoes
2 limes or lemons

Line 4 plates with lettuce or spinach leaves. Combine shrimp, scallops, celery, green onion, parsley, and lemon or lime juice in a medium bowl. Spoon a mound of shrimp mixture on top of lettuce. Place cucumber and cherry tomatoes on the side. Cut limes or lemons into wedges; place on plates. Let each person squeeze wedges over salad as desired. Makes 4 main dish servings.

Each serving contains:

Cal	Prot	Carb	Fib	Tot. Fat	Sat. Fat	Chol	Sodium
96	15g	7g	2g	1g	0g	74mg	177mg

Chicken, Peach, and Berry Salad

Peaches and berries say summer is here. Fresh berries turn leftover chicken into a delicious main-dish salad.

1 bunch spinach
1 celery stalk, sliced
2 fresh peaches, peeled, sliced
1 cup cubed cooked chicken
1 cup fresh raspberries or strawberries
2 tablespoons toasted walnuts
1/2 cup Honey–Poppy Seed Dressing, page 105

Thoroughly rinse spinach. Pat dry and tear into bite-size pieces. In salad bowl, combine spinach, celery, peaches, chicken, berries, and walnuts. Add dressing and toss gently to coat.

Or line 6 salad plates with spinach; arrange celery, peaches, and chicken on top. Scatter berries over top and drizzle with dressing. Sprinkle with walnuts. Makes 6 main dish servings.

Each serving contains:

Cal	Prot	Carb	Fib	Tot. Fat	Sat. Fat	Chol	Sodium
256	10g	34g	4g	11g	1g	20mg	69mg

Dressings and Sauces

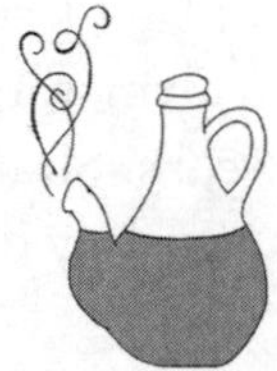

Although a beautiful salad or entrée may seem complete in itself, look again: A complementary dressing or sauce often adds the finishing touch and makes the ordinary memorable. This chapter will give you many ideas to choose from. Please add dressing and sauces sparingly. Nothing is worse than delicate salad greens wilted under too much dressing. Pasta, too, should be lightly sauced, not buried under a huge amount of sauce. A little goes a long way!

Olive oil adds a wonderful dimension to many sauces and dressings. Embraced by health-minded cooks worldwide, this mostly monounsaturated fat increases the amount of HDL (the "good" cholesterol) in the bloodstream, thereby helping to reduce the risk of heart disease. Use olive oil sparingly, because, like any fat, it is high in calories. Flavors vary among the various oils. Some are very mild; others are robust. In general, I recommend starting with the mild light-colored olive oils and working up to the deeper-flavored virgin oils.

Bring excitement to otherwise plain food by using sauces in new ways. Spinach-Walnut Pesto tastes great on pasta, but try using it as a flavorful sandwich spread, too. Choose any of the vinaigrettes to marinate cooked vegetables; then add the vegetables to your salad or serve them as a side dish. Your reputation as a creative cook will be made!

HOMEMADE VINEGARS

Leftover wine and very ripe fruits and berries can take on a new life as flavored vinegar. It is easy to make this gourmet item yourself. Low in calories, with no fat, vinegars add a healthful accent to salads and steamed vegetables or when sprinkled over fresh fruit.

Wine vinegar. Add 1 tablespoon distilled or cider vinegar to about 1 cup wine to create wine vinegar instantly.

Fruit or berry vinegar. Place 1 cup very ripe berries in a jar with 1-1/2 cups wine or distilled vinegar; cover and place in a cool dark cabinet for about three weeks. Strain liquid into a clean jar and discard pulp, and your vinegar is ready to enjoy.

Balsamic Herb Dressing

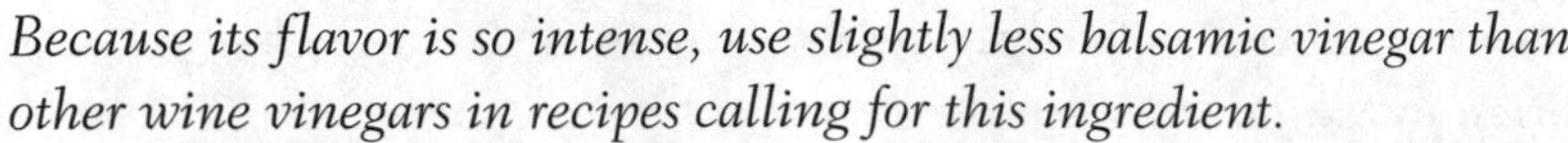

Because its flavor is so intense, use slightly less balsamic vinegar than other wine vinegars in recipes calling for this ingredient.

- 3 tablespoons balsamic vinegar
- 2 tablespoons fresh lemon juice
- 6 tablespoons olive oil
- 3 garlic cloves, crushed
- 1/2 teaspoon dry mustard
- 1/2 teaspoon dried-leaf basil
- 1/2 teaspoon dried-leaf oregano
- 1/2 teaspoon sweet paprika

Combine all ingredients in a jar with a tight-fitting lid and stir briskly with a fork. Or blend ingredients in a food processor or blender. Store in a covered container. Shake salad dressing vigorously before using. Makes about 2/3 cup.

Each tablespoon contains:

Cal	Prot	Carb	Fib	Tot. Fat	Sat. Fat	Chol	Sodium
71	0g	1g	0g	7g	1g	0mg	1mg

French Dressing

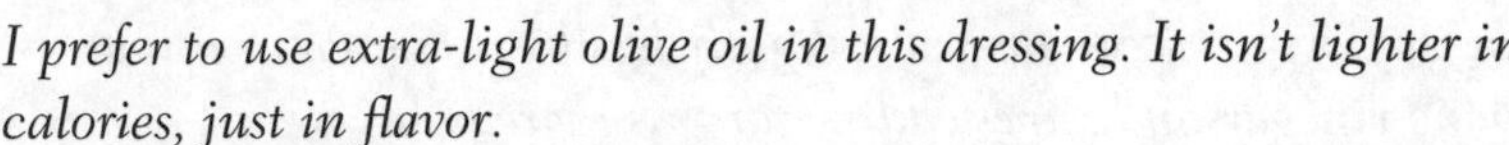

I prefer to use extra-light olive oil in this dressing. It isn't lighter in calories, just in flavor.

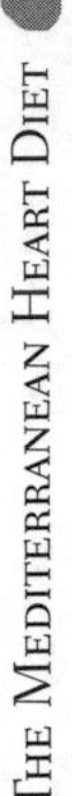

1/2 cup extra-light olive oil or canola oil
1/4 cup cider vinegar
2 tablespoons grated onion
2 tablespoons sugar
1/3 cup catsup
1 teaspoon sweet paprika
1 teaspoon black pepper
1 tablespoon fresh lemon juice
1/2 teaspoon Dijon mustard
2 garlic cloves, peeled

Place all ingredients in a blender and blend until well mixed. Pour into container and cover. Chill before using. Shake vigorously before pouring on salad greens. Makes about 1-1/4 cups.

Each tablespoon contains:

Cal	Prot	Carb	Fib	Tot. Fat	Sat. Fat	Chol	Sodium
59	0g	3g	0g	5g	0g	0mg	52mg

Honey–Poppy Seed Dressing

Drizzle a bit of this dressing over fresh fruit—it's a delightful way to enjoy your favorite fruits.

1/2 cup honey
1 tablespoon grated lemon zest
1/2 cup fresh lemon juice
3 tablespoons extra-light olive oil or canola oil
2 teaspoons poppy seeds

Combine honey, lemon zest, lemon juice, and oil in a small bowl. Stir in poppy seeds. Stir again before using. Makes about 1 cup.

Each tablespoon contains:

Cal	Prot	Carb	Fib	Tot. Fat	Sat. Fat	Chol	Sodium
59	0g	10g	0g	3g	0g	0mg	1mg

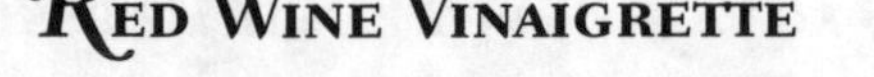

Red Wine Vinaigrette

Make a double recipe and use half as a marinade for cooked vegetables.

1/3 cup olive or canola oil
1/4 cup red wine vinegar
1 teaspoon sugar
1 teaspoon dry mustard
1/2 teaspoon sweet paprika
1 garlic clove, chopped

Combine all ingredients in a jar or container with a tight-fitting lid. Let stand at room temperature at least 2 hours. Shake vigorously before using. Makes about 2/3 cup.

Each tablespoon contains:

Cal	Prot	Carb	Fib	Tot. Fat	Sat. Fat	Chol	Sodium
63	0g	1g	0g	7g	0g	0mg	0mg

Italian Dressing

Just the right dressing to sprinkle over sliced tomatoes.

1/2 cup olive oil
2 tablespoons cider vinegar
2 tablespoons fresh lemon juice
1 garlic clove, minced
1 green onion, chopped
1/2 teaspoon dried-leaf oregano
1/2 teaspoon dry mustard
2 tablespoons unsalted tomato juice

Combine all ingredients in a jar or container with a tight-fitting lid. Shake and let stand at room temperature 1 hour before using. Shake vigorously before using. Makes about 1 cup.

Each tablespoon contains:

Cal	Prot	Carb	Fib	Tot. Fat	Sat. Fat	Chol	Sodium
62	0g	1g	0g	7g	1g	0mg	0mg

Basil–Blue Cheese Vinaigrette

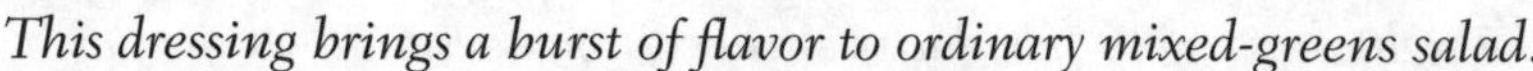

This dressing brings a burst of flavor to ordinary mixed-greens salad.

1/4 cup white wine vinegar or fresh lemon juice
3/4 cup olive oil
2 garlic cloves, minced
1/4 teaspoon dry mustard
1 teaspoon dried-leaf basil
1 teaspoon capers, drained
1/4 cup crumbled Roquefort or Gorgonzola cheese
Salt and pepper, to taste

In a small bowl, combine all ingredients. Cover and refrigerate at least 1 hour for flavors to blend. Makes about 1-1/2 cups.

Each tablespoon contains:

Cal	Prot	Carb	Fib	Tot. Fat	Sat. Fat	Chol	Sodium
66	0g	0g	0g	7g	1g	1mg	43mg

Cucumber-Yogurt Dressing

Make this cool and refreshing dressing early in the day and let the flavor develop. Spoon over fresh, ripe tomato slices.

1 cucumber, peeled, seeded, shredded
1/2 cup plain fat-free yogurt
2 tablespoons pine nuts
2 tablespoons capers, drained
1 tablespoon fresh lemon juice
1/2 teaspoon garlic powder
1 tablespoon chopped fresh parsley
Salt and pepper, to taste

In a small bowl, combine shredded cucumber with remaining ingredients. Cover and chill before serving. Makes about 1-1/4 cups.

Each tablespoon contains:

Cal	Prot	Carb	Fib	Tot. Fat	Sat. Fat	Chol	Sodium
9	1g	1g	0g	0g	0g	0mg	44mg

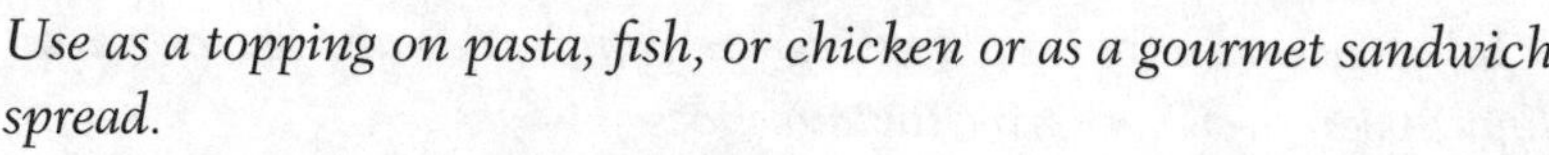

Spinach-Walnut Pesto

Use as a topping on pasta, fish, or chicken or as a gourmet sandwich spread.

1 cup packed fresh spinach leaves
2 garlic cloves, peeled
1/2 cup chopped walnuts
2 tablespoons olive oil
1/4 cup grated Parmesan cheese
1/4 cup plain fat-free yogurt
2 tablespoons Yogurt Cream Cheese, page 62
3 tablespoons fresh lemon juice
1/4 teaspoon grated nutmeg
1 tablespoon chopped fresh chives
Salt and pepper, to taste

Combine all ingredients in a food processor or blender. Process until thoroughly blended. It will be necessary to stop the machine a few times and scrape mixture down from the sides. Refrigerate in a container with a tight-fitting lid. Bring to room temperature and stir well before serving. Makes about 1-1/2 cups.

Each tablespoon contains:

Cal	Prot	Carb	Fib	Tot. Fat	Sat. Fat	Chol	Sodium
34	1g	1g	0g	3g	1g	1mg	35mg

Yogurt-Tomato Sauce

If ripe tomatoes are not available, use well-drained canned tomatoes.

2 large tomatoes, peeled, seeded, chopped
1/4 green bell pepper, chopped
3 tablespoons chopped fresh parsley
1/2 cup plain fat-free yogurt
1 green onion, chopped

In a small bowl, combine all ingredients. Cover and refrigerate at least 1 hour for flavors to blend. Makes about 1 cup.

Each tablespoon contains:

Cal	Prot	Carb	Fib	Tot. Fat	Sat. Fat	Chol	Sodium
9	1g	2g	0g	0g	0g	0mg	12mg

Corn-Tomato Sauce

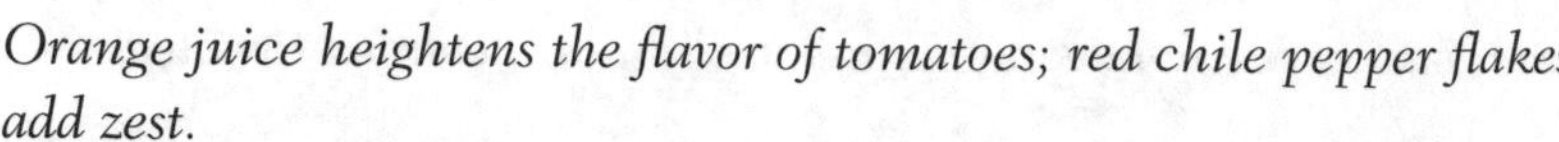

Orange juice heightens the flavor of tomatoes; red chile pepper flakes add zest.

4 cups chopped tomatoes
1 onion, chopped
1 green bell pepper, chopped
1 red bell pepper, chopped
1 fresh red chile pepper, chopped
1 tablespoon sugar
1/2 teaspoon salt
1/4 teaspoon ground ginger
1/4 teaspoon grated nutmeg
1-1/4 cups fresh orange juice
1 (17-oz.) can whole-kernel corn, drained
1/2 teaspoon red chile pepper flakes (optional)

In a 3-quart nonstick saucepan, combine all ingredients except corn and chile flakes, if using. Cook over medium heat, stirring occasionally, about 30 minutes. Add corn and chile pepper flakes, if using; cook 5 minutes. Makes about 6 cups.

Each 1/4 cup contains:

Cal	Prot	Carb	Fib	Tot. Fat	Sat. Fat	Chol	Sodium
33	1g	7g	1g	0g	0g	0mg	111mg

Red Bell Pepper Sauce

Jarred, roasted red bell peppers may be substituted for fresh.

2 red bell peppers, roasted, seeded, skinned, chopped
2 green onions, chopped
2 tablespoons chopped fresh parsley
1 tablespoon olive oil
1 garlic clove, minced
1 cup chopped fresh tomatoes

In a small bowl, combine all ingredients. Cover and refrigerate at least 20 minutes before serving. Serve as a topping on broiled fish or chicken or as a relish. Makes about 2 cups.

Each 1/4 cup contains:

Cal	Prot	Carb	Fib	Tot. Fat	Sat. Fat	Chol	Sodium
26	0g	2g	1g	2g	0g	0mg	55mg

Tomato Salsa

A versatile topping that is especially good with any egg dish.

1 (8-oz.) can low-sodium tomato sauce
1/4 cup chopped onion
2/3 cup chopped mild green chile peppers
1/4 to 1/2 teaspoon chili powder
2 tomatoes, chopped
1 tablespoon chopped fresh cilantro

Combine all ingredients in a small container. Cover and refrigerate. Let flavor develop 2 to 3 hours before using. Makes about 2 cups.

Each tablespoon contains:

Cal	Prot	Carb	Fib	Tot. Fat	Sat. Fat	Chol	Sodium
6	0g	1g	0g	0g	0g	0mg	2mg

Marinara Sauce

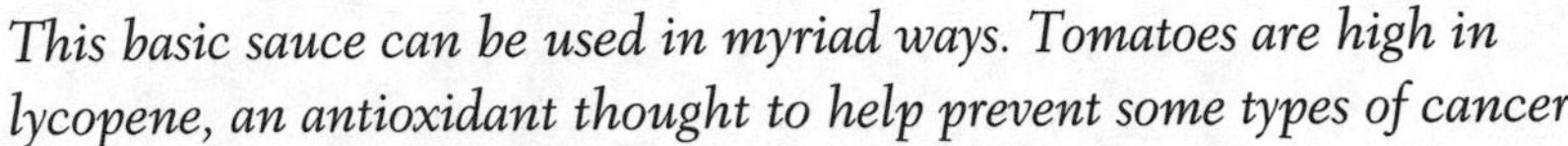

This basic sauce can be used in myriad ways. Tomatoes are high in lycopene, an antioxidant thought to help prevent some types of cancer.

3 tablespoons olive oil
1 cup chopped onion
2 garlic cloves, minced
1 (8-oz.) can low-sodium tomato sauce
2 fresh tomatoes, seeded, chopped
1/2 teaspoon sugar
2 tablespoons chopped fresh parsley
2 teaspoons dried-leaf basil
1 teaspoon dried-leaf oregano
Salt and pepper, to taste

In a medium saucepan, heat oil over medium heat. Add onion and garlic and sauté until onion is softened. Add remaining ingredients and bring to a boil. Reduce heat and simmer 15 minutes, stirring occasionally. Makes about 2 cups.

Each 1/4 cup contains:

Cal	Prot	Carb	Fib	Tot. Fat	Sat. Fat	Chol	Sodium
72	1g	6g	1g	5g	1g	0mg	44mg

Grains, Beans, and Pasta

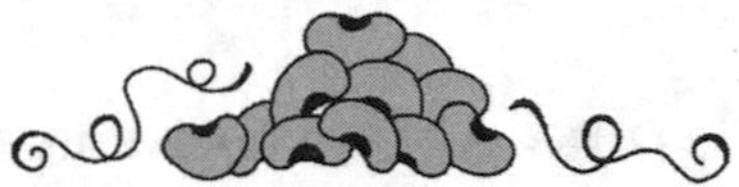

Beans and grains of all sorts play an important role in the foods of the Mediterranean. They are prepared in myriad ways and consumed in quantity every day—a practice that all of us would do well to follow. Meats, by contrast, are deemphasized and are used mainly to impart flavor. Mediterranean cooks also rely on vegetables, herbs, and nuts to provide delicious flavors in their bean and grain dishes.

Beans are used fresh, dried, or canned as a main ingredient in soups, stews, and salads and in pasta dishes. (Rinse canned beans with water and drain to reduce the sodium content.) If you have not made beans a part of your daily diet yet, start now! Your reward will be a more healthful diet as well as delicious food.

Pasta is versatile and nutritious, and it combines well with other foods. It is especially popular among those who want to increase the carbohydrates in their diet. It's delicious served hot or cold.

Pasta is made in a wide variety of shapes and sizes; a good rule is to serve light sauces on fine pasta and heavy or meat sauces on larger shapes such as ziti or penne. Sauce pasta lightly, as the Italians do; don't hide it under too much sauce.

Polenta is another popular food in the Mediterranean region. Made from coarse-grained cornmeal, polenta can be prepared easily

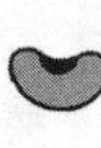

and enjoyed plain or accented with vegetable or meat sauces. Couscous, a precooked granular form of semolina that comes from North Africa, is a versatile cooking ingredient. Instant couscous, available in most supermarkets, can be prepared in a matter of minutes, an extremely useful attribute for busy cooks. Rice is another nutritious, filling carbohydrate that is versatile to cook with. For a special occasion, serve Saffron Rice. Saffron turns humble rice into a truly memorable meal.

Cooking Dried Beans

When using dried beans, presoaking before cooking is a must. Choose from two presoaking methods to shorten the cooking time for dried beans. In the first method, place the beans in a large bowl or pan. Add enough water to cover beans by 2 to 3 inches. Cover the pan or bowl and soak the beans for 8 hours.

As an alternative, place the beans in a large pot and cover with water. Bring water to a boil and boil 2 minutes. Cover the pot, remove from heat, and let stand 1 hour. Drain water and replace with fresh water. Return to heat. Simmer until beans are tender.

After presoaking the beans, cook them as your recipe directs. Cooking time for dried beans depends on the type and the age of the bean. Beans that have been stored for several months require a longer cooking time.

Rice and Fruit Salad

This chilled rice salad bursts with flavor and nutrition. Yogurt and orange juice combine to make an unusually good dressing.

2 cups cooked white rice
1 celery stalk, chopped
4 dried figs, chopped
2 dried apricots, chopped
1 cup seedless green grapes
1/2 cup orange low-fat yogurt
1/4 cup orange juice
1 orange, chopped, peeled
2 tablespoons chopped pistachios
2 tablespoons chopped fresh mint

In a large bowl, toss together rice, celery, figs, apricots, and grapes. In a cup, stir together orange yogurt and orange juice. Pour over rice mixture and stir to combine. Garnish with orange and chopped pistachios and fresh mint. Cover and refrigerate until chilled. Makes 6 servings.

Each serving contains:

Cal	Prot	Carb	Fib	Tot. Fat	Sat. Fat	Chol	Sodium
175	4g	37g	3g	2g	0g	1mg	23mg

Saffron Rice

If saffron is not available, substitute 3/4 teaspoon turmeric to achieve the golden color; however, the flavor will be different.

1/4 teaspoon saffron threads
1/4 cup hot water
1-3/4 cups reduced-sodium canned chicken broth
1 cup long-grain white rice
1 carrot, finely grated
2 green onions, chopped
1/4 cup chopped yellow bell pepper
Salt and pepper, to taste

In a cup, soak saffron threads in 1/4 cup hot water. Set aside for 20 minutes. Pour broth, saffron, and soaking water into a saucepan. Stir in rice and carrot and bring broth to a boil. Cover and reduce heat to simmer. Cook until liquid is absorbed, about 20 minutes. Stir in green onions and bell pepper. Season with salt and pepper, cover, and let stand 5 minutes. Serve at once. Makes 6 servings.

Each serving contains:

Cal	Prot	Carb	Fib	Tot. Fat	Sat. Fat	Chol	Sodium
134	4g	27g	1g	1g	0g	0mg	282mg

Beans, Rice, and Vegetables

Create a colorful side dish or satisfying vegetarian main dish with these ever-popular ingredients.

2 teaspoons olive oil
1 garlic clove, minced
1 cup chopped onion
1/4 cup diced celery
3/4 cup chopped red bell pepper
3/4 cup long-grain white rice
2 tomatoes, peeled, chopped
2 cups reduced-sodium canned chicken broth
1/2 teaspoon dried-leaf oregano
1/2 teaspoon dried-leaf marjoram
1/2 cup canned kidney beans
1/4 cup frozen green peas
Salt and pepper, to taste

Heat oil in a large saucepan over medium heat. Add garlic, onion, and celery and sauté until golden brown. Add bell pepper and cook 1 or 2 minutes. Stir in rice. Add tomatoes and chicken broth to rice with oregano and marjoram. Cover, reduce heat to low, and simmer 20 minutes or until broth is absorbed.

Meanwhile, rinse beans and drain again; set aside. Stir peas and beans into rice mixture; cover and set aside 5 minutes. Season with salt and pepper. Fluff mixture with a fork before serving. Makes 4 servings.

Each serving contains:

Cal	Prot	Carb	Fib	Tot. Fat	Sat. Fat	Chol	Sodium
248	9g	45g	6g	4g	1g	0mg	477mg

Walnut Pilaf

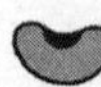

You may also use other nuts, such as almonds, pine nuts, or hazelnuts.

2 teaspoons olive oil
1 onion, chopped
1 cup long-grain white rice
1/4 cup Zante currants or chopped raisins
1 cup vermicelli, broken in 1-inch pieces
2 1/2 cups water or reduced-sodium canned chicken broth
1/4 cup chopped walnuts

Heat oil in a large saucepan over medium heat. Add onion and rice and sauté, stirring, until rice is coated. Add remaining ingredients, except walnuts. Bring to a boil; reduce heat. Cover and cook about 20 minutes until rice is tender and liquid is absorbed. Stir in walnuts, cover, and set aside for 5 minutes. Fluff mixture with a fork before serving. Makes 6 servings.

Each serving contains:

Cal	Prot	Carb	Fib	Tot. Fat	Sat. Fat	Chol	Sodium
252	6g	46g	2g	5g	1g	0mg	6mg

Variation
Walnut-Chicken Casserole

Add 1/2 cup cooked green peas and 1 cup chopped cooked chicken with the walnuts.

Spicy Cannellini Beans

A simple can of beans can be the start of a delicious main dish or side dish.

2 (16-oz.) cans cannellini (white kidney) beans, drained
1 teaspoon olive oil
2 garlic cloves, minced
1/4 onion, chopped
1 tablespoon chopped fresh parsley
1 teaspoon dry mustard
Dash red chile pepper flakes

Rinse beans and drain again; set aside. Heat oil in a nonstick skillet over medium heat. Add garlic and onion and sauté until softened. Add all remaining ingredients; simmer, stirring, about 5 minutes. Makes 4 servings.

Each serving contains:

Cal	Prot	Carb	Fib	Tot. Fat	Sat. Fat	Chol	Sodium
194	9g	33g	9g	2g	0g	0mg	472mg

Green Beans with Sage

Wine and fresh sage bring unexpected flavor to this easy-to-make dish.

1 lb. fresh green beans, trimmed and cut in 1-inch pieces
1 onion, sliced crosswise, separated in rings
1/2 cup reduced-sodium canned beef broth
1/2 cup vermouth or white wine
1 tablespoon chopped pimiento
1 tablespoon chopped fresh sage or 1 teaspoon dried
1 tablespoon grated lemon peel
1/2 teaspoon sweet paprika
Salt and pepper, to taste

Preheat oven to 350°F (175°C). In a baking dish, layer green beans and onion rings. Combine remaining ingredients and pour over vegetables. Cover and bake about 40 minutes. Uncover and bake 10 minutes longer, or until vegetables are tender. Makes 4 servings.

Each serving contains:

Cal	Prot	Carb	Fib	Tot. Fat	Sat. Fat	Chol	Sodium
87	3g	13g	2g	0g	0g	0mg	184mg

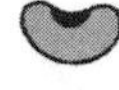

Macaroni Frittata

Turn that bit of extra pasta into a delightful entrée.

4 eggs or 1 cup egg substitute
1 tablespoon cornstarch
1 tablespoon capers, drained
6 or 7 pitted black olives, sliced
1 tablespoon chopped fresh parsley
1 tablespoon olive oil
2 tablespoons butter
1/4 medium onion, chopped
1/2 cup chopped red bell pepper
1 cup cooked macaroni or other small pasta
Salt and black pepper, to taste
2 tomatoes, seeded, chopped
Chopped fresh basil

Preheat broiler. In a medium bowl, beat eggs or egg substitute and cornstarch. Stir in capers, olives, and parsley; set aside. In a 10-inch nonstick fry pan with a flameproof handle, heat oil and butter over medium heat. Add onion and bell pepper and sauté until softened. Add macaroni and season with salt and black pepper. Stir together until heated. Remove from heat.

Pour egg mixture evenly over mixture in skillet. Reduce heat to low, cover and cook 5 to 7 minutes. Remove cover and place fry pan under broiler for 5 minutes or until top is firm and slightly browned. Loosen edges and cut into wedges. Top each wedge with tomatoes and basil. Makes 6 servings.

Each serving contains:

Cal	Prot	Carb	Fib	Tot. Fat	Sat. Fat	Chol	Sodium
161	5g	12g	2g	11g	4g	152mg	175mg

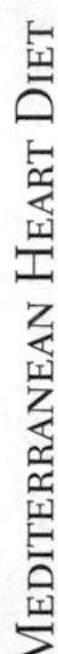

Spaghetti with Italian Sausage–Tomato Sauce

No one will suspect that you made this dish so quickly and easily!

1 lb. sweet Italian sausage links
1/4 onion, chopped
1/4 teaspoon dried-leaf basil
1/4 teaspoon dried-leaf oregano
1/4 teaspoon dried-leaf marjoram
1 (28-oz.) can whole tomatoes, chopped, with juice
1 (8-oz.) can low-sodium tomato sauce
3 cups cooked spaghetti
Fresh chopped parsley
1/4 cup grated Romano cheese

Slit sausage open and remove casing; crumble or slice sausage. In a 12-inch nonstick sauté pan, brown sausage over medium heat; drain excess fat. Add onion and sauté until softened. Add basil, oregano, marjoram, tomatoes with juice, and tomato sauce. Cover and cook about 20 minutes. Meanwhile, cook spaghetti according to package directions and drain. Spoon sausage and sauce over hot spaghetti. Sprinkle with chopped parsley and Romano cheese. Makes 6 servings.

Each serving contains:

Cal	Prot	Carb	Fib	Tot. Fat	Sat. Fat	Chol	Sodium
416	17g	30g	3g	26g	10g	62mg	804mg

Savory Crêpes

Fill with Ricotta Cheese Filling, on page 128, or your favorite filling.

4 eggs
1-1/2 cups water
1-1/2 cups all-purpose flour
2 tablespoons canola oil
1/4 teaspoon salt (optional)

Combine all ingredients in a medium bowl, blender, or food processor; mix until well blended. Let batter rest about 30 minutes.

Lightly brush a 6- to 7-inch crêpe pan with oil and heat pan over medium heat. Pour about 2 tablespoons batter into pan; immediately tilt pan so batter flows over the bottom. Cook until surface looks dry and edges are lacy and brown. (Only 1 side needs to be cooked.) Place each crêpe on a plate to cool; place waxed paper between crêpes. Makes 28 crêpes.

Each crêpe contains:

Cal	Prot	Carb	Fib	Tot. Fat	Sat. Fat	Chol	Sodium
44	2g	5g	0g	2g	0g	31mg	10mg

Manicotti with Ricotta Cheese Filling

This recipe makes two large pans of filled manicotti, enough for a party—or serve one now and freeze the other.

Ricotta Cheese Filling:
- 2 cups ricotta cheese
- 1/4 cup grated Parmesan cheese
- 1 egg
- 1 cup shredded mozzarella cheese
- 3 tablespoons chopped fresh parsley
- 1 tablespoon chopped fresh basil
- 1/4 teaspoon grated nutmeg
- Salt and pepper, to taste

Savory Crêpes, page 127
Marinara Sauce, page 115
1/4 cup grated Parmesan cheese, for garnish

Preheat oven to 375°F (190°C). In medium bowl, stir together all filling ingredients. Spoon about 1/4 cup filling down center of each crêpe. Roll to enclose filling and place, seam side down, in 2 shallow baking dishes.

Spoon Marinara Sauce over the center of filled crêpes. Sprinkle with Parmesan cheese. Bake about 20 minutes, or until hot and bubbly. Makes 14 (two-crêpe) servings.

Each serving contains:

Cal	Prot	Carb	Fib	Tot. Fat	Sat. Fat	Chol	Sodium
234	11g	15g	1g	14g	6g	103mg	196mg

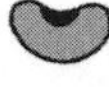

Penne Pasta Primavera

When you team a colorful medley of springtime vegetables with pasta, dinner is served in 30 minutes.

2 teaspoons olive oil
3 asparagus spears, peeled, cut in 2-inch pieces
1 zucchini, halved lengthwise, sliced crosswise
1 yellow bell pepper, cut in strips
2 garlic cloves, minced
1/4 onion, sliced crosswise
1/4 cup reduced-sodium canned chicken broth
1 teaspoon dried-leaf thyme
1 teaspoon dried-leaf oregano
1 tablespoon chopped fresh parsley
1 (16-oz.) package penne pasta
12 cherry tomatoes, halved
Salt and pepper, to taste

Heat oil in a 10-inch fry pan over medium heat. Add asparagus, zucchini, bell pepper, garlic, and onion; sauté 5 minutes, stirring occasionally. Add chicken broth, thyme, oregano, and parsley; cover and cook 5 minutes.

Meanwhile, cook pasta according to package directions and drain. Toss pasta, sautéed vegetables, and tomatoes together. Season with salt and pepper. Serve warm or chilled. Makes 8 servings.

Each serving contains:

Cal	Prot	Carb	Fib	Tot. Fat	Sat. Fat	Chol	Sodium
259	9g	50g	4g	2g	0g	0mg	66mg

Linguine with Mushroom, Basil, and Sun-Dried Tomato Sauce

A little evaporated milk dramatically changes the color and flavor of this sauce.

1 tablespoon olive oil
1/2 onion, sliced
1 green bell pepper, sliced
1 cup sliced fresh mushrooms
1/2 cup low-fat evaporated milk
1/2 cup reduced-sodium canned chicken broth
3 tablespoons shredded fresh basil
1/4 cup oil-pack sun-dried tomatoes, chopped
3 cups cooked linguine
Grated Parmesan cheese (optional)

In large saucepan over medium heat, heat oil. Add onion, bell pepper, and mushrooms and sauté until softened. Stir in evaporated milk and chicken broth; bring to a boil. Reduce heat and simmer until liquid is slightly reduced, about 5 minutes. Add basil and sun-dried tomatoes. Cook about 2 minutes more. Place cooked pasta in a bowl and toss with sauce. Sprinkle each serving with grated Parmesan cheese, if desired. Makes 6 servings.

Each serving contains:

Cal	Prot	Carb	Fib	Tot. Fat	Sat. Fat	Chol	Sodium
157	7g	22g	2g	5g	2g	6mg	160mg

Fettuccine with Herbs and Walnuts

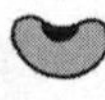

This is one of my most requested recipes, which I often serve to guests. It is excellent as a main dish or as a side dish for grilled meats. Fine egg noodles are a good substitute for the fettuccine.

2 tablespoons olive oil
1 tablespoon butter
1/4 cup minced fresh parsley
2 teaspoons dried-leaf oregano
2 teaspoons dried-leaf basil
1 teaspoon dried-leaf rosemary
2 garlic cloves, minced
3 tablespoons toasted walnuts
Salt and pepper, to taste
1/2 lb. fettuccine, cooked
2 tablespoons grated Parmesan cheese

In a small skillet, heat oil, butter, parsley, oregano, basil, rosemary, and garlic. Cook over low heat about 2 minutes. Remove from heat; stir in walnuts and season with salt and pepper.

In a large serving dish, combine hot fettuccine, herb-walnut mixture, and Parmesan cheese. Toss gently to combine. Serve at once. Makes 4 servings.

Each serving contains:

Cal	Prot	Carb	Fib	Tot. Fat	Sat. Fat	Chol	Sodium
224	6g	19g	2g	14g	4g	10mg	135mg

Zucchini and Garbanzo Beans Provençal

Tender, fresh zucchini in a simple sauce makes an easy main dish.

1 tablespoon olive oil
1/2 large onion, chopped
2 large garlic cloves, minced
1 teaspoon dried-leaf basil
1/4 teaspoon dried-leaf oregano
1 (28-oz.) can chopped Italian tomatoes, with juice
1/4 cup red wine
1/4 cup unsalted tomato paste
1/2 cup water
1/2 lb. pasta
1 lb. zucchini, sliced
1 (15-oz.) can garbanzo beans (chickpeas), drained and rinsed
3 tablespoons grated Parmesan cheese
Salt and pepper, to taste

Heat oil in a skillet over medium heat. Add onion, garlic, basil, and oregano; sauté 2 to 3 minutes. Add tomatoes with juice, wine, tomato paste, and water. Cover, reduce heat to low, and simmer 15 to 20 minutes. Add zucchini and beans to tomato sauce, cover, and simmer until zucchini is tender, 10 to 15 minutes.

Meanwhile, cook pasta according to package directions, omitting salt, and drain. In a large bowl, combine tomato sauce and pasta. Sprinkle with cheese and season with salt and pepper. Makes 6 servings.

Each serving contains:

Cal	Prot	Carb	Fib	Tot. Fat	Sat. Fat	Chol	Sodium
159	8g	23g	6g	4g	1g	2mg	474mg

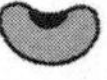

Polenta with Tomato and Fontina

Polenta is usually served topped with stewed meat, a sauce, or cheese.

4 cups reduced-sodium canned chicken broth or water
1/2 teaspoon salt
1 cup coarse cornmeal
1 tomato, peeled, seeded, chopped
1 tablespoon chopped fresh parsley
1 tablespoon minced green onion
1/4 teaspoon garlic powder
1/4 cup grated Fontina cheese

In a large pan, bring chicken broth or water and salt to a boil. Stirring constantly, gradually add cornmeal. Cook, stirring with a long-handled wooden spoon over medium heat until thickened, about 20 minutes. (Caution: Polenta can spatter.) Stir in remaining ingredients. Serve at once or pour into a flat baking dish and let cool. Slice and reheat to serve. Makes 6 servings.

Each serving contains:

Cal	Prot	Carb	Fib	Tot. Fat	Sat. Fat	Chol	Sodium
129	7g	20g	2g	3g	1g	5mg	749mg

COUSCOUS WITH CHICKEN AND DRIED APRICOTS

Make this North African–style dish in minutes.

1 (10-oz.) package couscous
1 cup reduced-sodium canned chicken broth
1/4 teaspoon turmeric
1 tablespoon fresh lemon juice
1/2 cup chopped dried apricots
1 cup cubed cooked chicken
1/4 red or yellow bell pepper, chopped
2 tablespoons chopped roasted almonds

Cook couscous according to package directions, using chicken broth and turmeric in place of water. Add remaining ingredients and stir to combine. Makes 4 servings.

Each serving contains:

Cal	Prot	Carb	Fib	Tot. Fat	Sat. Fat	Chol	Sodium
435	26g	69g	6g	8g	2g	31mg	232mg

Lentils with Vegetables

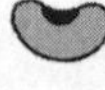

The right seasoning mixture imparts rich flavor to bean or lentil dishes. Try this recipe and see for yourself!

1 cup dried lentils
1/2 onion, chopped
1/2 teaspoon ground cardamom
1 carrot, sliced
1/2 teaspoon black pepper
1 red bell pepper, sliced
1/2 teaspoon ground cinnamon
2 cups water or vegetable stock
1 (16-oz.) can chopped tomatoes
Salt and black pepper, to taste
Red chile pepper flakes (optional)

Rinse and sort lentils. In a 3-quart saucepan, combine all ingredients except salt, black pepper, and optional chile flakes. Bring to a boil. Cover, reduce heat, and simmer until lentils are tender, about 30 minutes. Season with salt, black pepper, and red chile pepper flakes, if desired. Makes 6 servings.

Each serving contains:

Cal	Prot	Carb	Fib	Tot. Fat	Sat. Fat	Chol	Sodium
127	9g	24g	8g	1g	0g	0mg	65mg

Barley, Mushroom, and Feta Casserole

Enjoy this hearty casserole as a side dish or a vegetarian main dish.

2 tablespoons olive oil
1/2 cup chopped celery
1 small onion, chopped
2 garlic cloves, chopped
1 cup pearl barley
3 cups water or reduced-sodium canned chicken broth
1 cup chopped fresh mushrooms
2 tablespoons chopped fresh basil or 2 teaspoons dried basil
1/2 cup frozen green peas
Salt and pepper, to taste
1/2 cup crumbled herbed feta cheese
2 tablespoons chopped walnuts

In a Dutch oven or heavy saucepan over medium heat, heat 1 tablespoon of the olive oil. Add celery, onion, and garlic and sauté until softened, stirring occasionally. Add barley and stir until coated. Pour in water or broth. Reduce heat to low, cover, and simmer about 50 minutes.

In a small skillet over medium heat, heat remaining 1 tablespoon oil; add mushrooms and cook until softened, about 5 minutes. Stir mushrooms, basil, and peas into barley mixture. Season with salt and pepper. Cover and cook 5 minutes longer. Spoon into serving dish and top with cheese and walnuts. Or place in an ovenproof dish and broil until cheese melts. Makes 8 servings.

Each serving contains:

Cal	Prot	Carb	Fib	Tot. Fat	Sat. Fat	Chol	Sodium
174	5g	24g	5g	7g	2g	8mg	128mg

Spanish Rice and Beans

Serve as a side dish or as a bed for broiled fish or chicken.

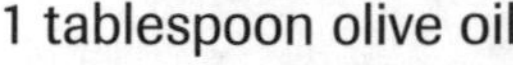

1 tablespoon olive oil
2 green onions, chopped
1 garlic clove, chopped
1 celery stalk, chopped
1 carrot, chopped
1 cup uncooked long-grain brown rice
3/4 cup water
1 (14-1/4-oz.) can diced tomatoes, with juice
1 (15-oz.) can pinto or pink kidney beans, drained
1 tablespoon chopped fresh mint or basil
Salt and pepper, to taste

Heat oil in a large saucepan over medium heat. Add green onions, garlic, celery, and carrot; sauté until softened. Add rice and stir to coat. Add water and tomatoes with juice. Cover pan, reduce heat to low, and simmer 40 to 45 minutes. Rinse and drain beans; add beans and mint or basil to rice mixture. Cover and cook until heated through and rice is tender, about 5 minutes. Season with salt and pepper, to taste. Makes 8 servings.

Each serving contains:

Cal	Prot	Carb	Fib	Tot. Fat	Sat. Fat	Chol	Sodium
164	6g	30g	5g	3g	0g	0mg	218mg

Risotto with Sun-Dried Tomatoes and Artichokes

It takes a little time to prepare this traditional Italian dish, but the results are well worth it.

4 cups reduced-sodium canned chicken broth or water
1/2 cup white wine
1 tablespoon olive oil
4 green onions, chopped
1 cup arborio rice
1/2 cup fresh or frozen green peas
2 tablespoons chopped oil-pack sun-dried tomatoes
1/4 cup chopped marinated artichoke hearts, drained
1/4 cup grated Parmesan cheese
1 tablespoon chopped fresh parsley or basil

Combine broth or water and wine in a saucepan and bring to a simmer; keep broth simmering as it is used. Heat oil in a large skillet or saucepan over medium heat. Add green onions and rice, cook, stirring, until onions soften. Stir in 1/2 cup broth mixture; cook, stirring, until liquid is absorbed. Continue adding hot broth mixture 1/2 cup at a time after previous amount is absorbed, until all is used. Add peas, sun-dried tomatoes, and artichokes. Cook, stirring, 4 to 5 minutes. Total cooking time is 20 to 25 minutes; rice will become creamy. Add cheese and parsley or basil. Mix thoroughly and serve at once. Makes 8 side-dish servings.

Each serving contains:

Cal	Prot	Carb	Fib	Tot. Fat	Sat. Fat	Chol	Sodium
180	7g	26g	1g	4g	1g	2mg	478mg

Fish and Seafood

Fresh fish, like fresh vegetables, is an important part of the Mediterranean diet. If you live close to the sea, most likely you are able to purchase fresh whole fish. However, those who live away from coastal areas seem to prefer fillets. If you do not have access to the fresh catch of the day, don't despair. Modern processing at sea results in quick freezing, which helps preserve flavor and texture. If someone in your family likes to fish, encourage him or her to bring home the catch.

Because seafood is quick and easy to prepare, have it often. Include fish in your menus two or three times a week. For best results, always cook fish on high heat for a short time, because overcooking both toughens and dries out fish.

Besides wonderful flavor, as an added bonus when you eat fish, you get the benefits of omega-3—a very good fat. Herring, mackerel, salmon, trout, and tuna are some of the best sources of omega-3 fatty acids. These benefits can be diminished when the fish is deep-fried and heavily sauced with butter or cream. The most healthful way to prepare fish is to bake, broil, poach, stir-fry, or steam it.

During warm weather months, you might crave a cold dish for lunch; Shrimp, Beans, and Pasta will fill the bill. For a special occasion, Halibut with Citrus Sauce or Sole and Vegetables in Packets vie for the number-one choice. Tender Scallop and Vegetable

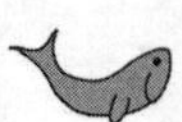

Kabobs taste so good that no one will suspect they were prepared in minutes.

People living in each of the countries bordering the Mediterranean Sea add their own embellishments to their seafood catch. The Spanish are fond of adding nuts, particularly almonds and hazelnuts, along with a variety of olives, for example. The Greeks and Italians frequently add fresh tomatoes to their fish dishes, while the French add a dash of vermouth and fresh tarragon leaves. Each combination is special, and each brings out the best flavors possible.

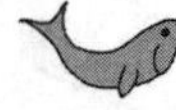

Spanish-Style Fish

Steamed rice and fresh fruit slices complete this meal.

1/2 cup dry bread crumbs
1/2 teaspoon dried-leaf thyme
1/4 teaspoon garlic powder
1 lb. sole or flounder fillets
1 egg, beaten
2 tablespoons olive oil
1 tablespoon butter
1 tablespoon fresh lemon juice
1/4 teaspoon red chile pepper flakes
2 tablespoons chopped roasted hazelnuts
1 tablespoon chopped fresh parsley

Combine bread crumbs, thyme, and garlic powder; set aside. Dip fillets in beaten egg, then into bread crumb mixture. Heat oil in a large skillet over medium heat and sauté fillets on both sides until golden. Place on a serving platter and keep warm.

Add butter to the skillet and heat until melted. Add lemon juice and remaining ingredients. Cook, stirring, until hot. Spoon over fillets and serve at once. Makes 4 servings.

Each serving contains:

Cal	Prot	Carb	Fib	Tot. Fat	Sat. Fat	Chol	Sodium
285	25g	11g	1g	15g	4g	115mg	225mg

Baked Cod and Tomatoes over Brown Rice

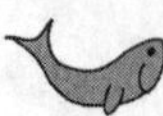

Always bake fish at high heat; this helps retain moisture.

1 lb. cod fillets
1 garlic clove, minced
1/2 teaspoon dried-leaf basil
Freshly ground black pepper to taste
1-1/2 cups diced fresh tomatoes
2 green onions, chopped
2 tablespoons chopped fresh parsley
2 cups cooked brown rice

Preheat oven to 425°F (220°C). Spray a baking dish with olive-oil cooking spray. Place fillets in single layer in baking dish and spray tops with olive-oil cooking spray. Sprinkle garlic, basil, and pepper over fish. Arrange tomatoes and green onions over fillets. Sprinkle with parsley. Cover with foil. Bake 10 to 15 minutes, or until fish flakes. Serve over hot rice. Makes 4 servings.

Each serving contains:

Cal	Prot	Carb	Fib	Tot. Fat	Sat. Fat	Chol	Sodium
220	24g	26g	3g	2g	0g	49mg	74mg

Halibut with Citrus Sauce

A mild-flavored fish combines beautifully with a tangy and flavorful sauce.

1/4 cup grapefruit juice
1/4 cup orange juice
1 teaspoon grated orange peel
1/4 cup raisins
1 green onion, chopped
1 lb. halibut fillets
1 tomato, sliced
1 orange, peeled, segmented

Spray a baking dish large enough to hold fillets in a single layer with olive-oil cooking spray. In a small mixing bowl, combine grapefruit juice, orange juice, orange peel, raisins, and green onion. Place fillets in prepared baking dish; pour juice mixture over fillets. Turn to coat both sides. Cover and refrigerate about 20 minutes.

Preheat oven to 425°F (220°C). Remove cover and top with tomato slices and orange segments. Spoon juice over tomatoes. Bake uncovered about 10 minutes, or until fish flakes. Makes 4 servings.

Each serving contains:

Cal	Prot	Carb	Fib	Tot. Fat	Sat. Fat	Chol	Sodium
190	25g	16g	2g	3g	1g	36mg	66mg

Poached Tuna Steaks

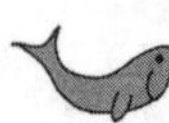

A broiled topping adds extra flair and flavor.

2 tablespoons fresh lemon juice
2 tablespoons celery leaves
1 bay leaf
1 quart water
1 lb. tuna steaks, about 1 inch thick
1/3 cup plain fat-free yogurt
3 tablespoons nonfat mayonnaise
2 teaspoons minced fresh chives
1/4 teaspoon salt
1/4 teaspoon pepper
1/4 teaspoon sweet paprika
Lemon wedges

Preheat broiler. In a 12-inch skillet, combine lemon juice, celery leaves, bay leaf, and water. Bring to a boil. Add tuna steaks; cover and simmer 4 minutes, or until barely cooked through.

With slotted spoon or spatula, carefully lift fish out of water; place on broiler pan. In a small bowl, combine yogurt, mayonnaise, chives, salt, pepper, and paprika. Spread over top of each steak. Broil 5 or 6 inches from heat until bubbly on top. Garnish with lemon wedges. Makes 4 servings.

Each serving contains:

Cal	Prot	Carb	Fib	Tot. Fat	Sat. Fat	Chol	Sodium
156	27g	9g	1g	1g	0g	54mg	396mg

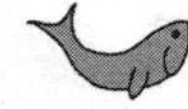

Cod Español

This cod dish is spicy, with wonderful character. Try it!

2 teaspoons olive oil
3 garlic cloves, chopped
1 onion, chopped
4 tomatoes (1 lb.), chopped
1 green or red bell pepper, chopped, or 1 green chile pepper, chopped
3 tablespoons chopped fresh parsley
1/2 teaspoon ground cinnamon
1 lb. cod, cut in 1-inch cubes
2 tablespoons toasted sliced almonds

Heat oil in a large skillet over medium heat. Add garlic and onion and sauté until softened. Add tomatoes, bell pepper or chile pepper, and parsley. Cook 3 to 4 minutes, stirring occasionally. Stir in cinnamon. Add cod, cover, and cook until cod flakes, about 10 minutes. Sprinkle with almonds. Makes 4 servings.

Each serving contains:

Cal	Prot	Carb	Fib	Tot. Fat	Sat. Fat	Chol	Sodium
184	23g	12g	3g	6g	1g	49mg	75mg

Sole and Vegetables in Packets

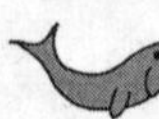

Packets are made of parchment or foil for no-mess baking.

1 carrot, julienned
1/2 onion, sliced in rings
2 (6-oz.) sole fillets
1/4 cup fresh lime juice
Sweet paprika
2 tablespoons sliced pimiento-stuffed olives
2 tablespoons chopped fresh parsley
2 teaspoons dried rosemary

Preheat oven to 425°F (220°C). Cook carrot in 1/2 cup boiling water in saucepan for 5 minutes. Drain and set aside.

Cut parchment or foil into pieces large enough to wrap each fillet. Place half of carrot strips and onion rings in center of each piece. Place 1 fillet on top of each vegetable portion. Pour lime juice over fillets and sprinkle with paprika. Scatter olives on top and sprinkle with parsley and rosemary. Fold parchment edges together and roll and fold to seal. Place on a baking sheet with a rim and bake 8 to 10 minutes. To serve, place each packet on plate, cut a slash on top, and tear open. Makes 2 servings.

Each serving contains:

Cal	Prot	Carb	Fib	Tot. Fat	Sat. Fat	Chol	Sodium
202	33g	10g	3g	3g	1g	82mg	320mg

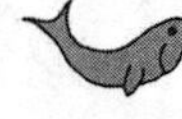

RED SNAPPER WITH WINE SAUCE

Red bell pepper, peas, and raisins add color and interest to this dish.

1 teaspoon olive oil
1 green onion, chopped
1/4 cup sliced red bell pepper
1 garlic clove, minced
2 tablespoons raisins
1/4 teaspoon ground cinnamon
3/4 cup white wine
1/2 cup frozen petite green peas
1 lb. red snapper fillets

In a skillet, heat oil over medium heat. Add green onion, bell pepper, and garlic and sauté until softened. Add raisins, cinnamon, wine, and peas. Rinse fillets and pat dry. Place in pan. Spoon wine mixture over fillets. Cover and simmer 5 minutes; remove cover. Spoon sauce over fish and simmer until fish just flakes, about 5 minutes. Serve with sauce. Makes 4 servings.

Each serving contains:

Cal	Prot	Carb	Fib	Tot. Fat	Sat. Fat	Chol	Sodium
178	24g	6g	1g	3g	1g	42mg	77mg

Yogurt-Topped Fillets

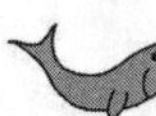

Tomato sauce and paprika add a blush of color to the creamy topping.

1/3 cup plain low-fat yogurt
1 tablespoon tomato sauce
1/2 teaspoon sweet paprika
1 tablespoon capers, drained
2 teaspoons chopped fresh parsley
3/4 lb. red snapper fillets

Preheat broiler. In a cup, mix yogurt, tomato sauce, paprika, capers, and parsley. Spray a broiling pan with olive-oil cooking spray. Place fillets on broiler pan; spread fillet tops with yogurt mixture. Broil without turning 6 to 8 minutes, or until fish flakes. Makes 4 servings.

Each serving contains:

Cal	Prot	Carb	Fib	Tot. Fat	Sat. Fat	Chol	Sodium
96	18g	2g	0g	1g	0g	32mg	130mg

Salmon with Rice and Beans

For a more festive dish, sprinkle chopped nuts over the parsley.

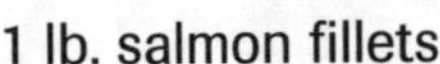

1 lb. salmon fillets
1 teaspoon olive oil
1 teaspoon dried-leaf oregano
1/2 recipe Spanish Rice and Beans, page 137
1 tablespoon chopped fresh parsley
Lemon wedges

Preheat broiler. Spray a broiler pan with olive-oil cooking spray. Rinse fillets and pat dry. Brush fillets with oil and sprinkle with oregano; broil about 10 minutes per inch of fish, until fish flakes. Serve with Spanish Rice and Beans. Garnish with parsley and lemon wedges. Serve at once. Makes 4 servings.

Each serving contains:

Cal	Prot	Carb	Fib	Tot. Fat	Sat. Fat	Chol	Sodium
279	27g	18g	4g	11g	2g	62mg	265mg

Sea Bass in Salsa

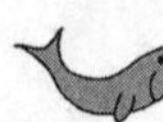

Achieve the level of hotness you prefer by selecting the mild bell pepper, Anaheim chile, or the hotter jalapeño chile.

1 cup chopped tomatoes
1/4 onion, chopped
1 green bell pepper, seeded, sliced
1/2 cup cooked lentils, drained
1/2 teaspoon dried-leaf oregano
Salt and pepper, to taste
1 lb. sea bass fillets

Spray a large fry pan with olive-oil cooking spray. Add tomatoes and onion. Cook, stirring, 3 to 5 minutes. Add bell pepper, lentils, oregano, salt, and pepper. Cook about 5 minutes longer. Rinse fillets and pat dry. Place fillets in a single layer in pan and spoon the tomato mixture on top. Cover and cook about 10 minutes, or until fish flakes. Serve at once. Makes 4 servings.

Each serving contains:

Cal	Prot	Carb	Fib	Tot. Fat	Sat. Fat	Chol	Sodium
159	24g	10g	3g	3g	1g	46mg	155mg

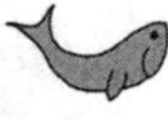

Sole Florentine

The creamed spinach filling is brightened by mushrooms and pimiento.

2 teaspoons olive oil
1/2 onion, chopped
1 garlic clove, minced
2 tablespoons all-purpose flour
1 cup fat-free milk
1/2 cup sliced fresh mushrooms
2 tablespoons pimiento, chopped
1/4 teaspoon grated nutmeg
1 (10-oz.) package frozen spinach, thawed, drained
1 lb. sole fillets
2 cups cooked barley

Preheat oven to 425°F (220°C). Spray a baking dish with olive-oil cooking spray. In a saucepan, heat oil over medium heat. Add onion and garlic and sauté until softened. Stir in flour and milk. Cook, stirring, until thickened. Stir in mushrooms, pimiento, nutmeg, and spinach. Thoroughly combine.

Spread mixture on fillets. Roll up and secure with wooden picks. Place in prepared baking dish. Cover and bake about 15 minutes, or until fish flakes. Serve with barley. Makes 4 servings.

Each serving contains:

Cal	Prot	Carb	Fib	Tot. Fat	Sat. Fat	Chol	Sodium
283	28g	33g	6g	4g	1g	56mg	178mg

Scallop and Vegetable Kabobs

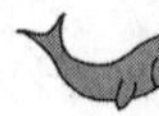

Italian Dressing is used as a marinade.

1 cup Italian Dressing, page 107
1 lb. scallops
1 small onion, quartered, leaves separated
1 red bell pepper, seeded, cut into small squares
12 small fresh mushrooms
1 green bell pepper, cut into small squares
2 cups cooked rice
1 tablespoon chopped fresh parsley

Pour Italian Dressing into a mixing bowl. Add scallops and onion; toss to coat all pieces. Cover and refrigerate at least 2 hours.

Preheat broiler. Alternate scallops, onion leaves, red bell pepper, mushrooms, and green bell pepper on metal skewers. Broil, turning often, about 7 minutes. Serve with rice, sprinkled with parsley. Makes 4 servings.

Each serving contains:

Cal	Prot	Carb	Fib	Tot. Fat	Sat. Fat	Chol	Sodium
486	23g	35g	3g	29g	4g	37mg	189mg

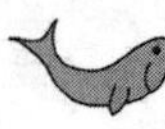

Clams in White Wine Sauce

The delicate flavor of clams is not overpowered by the sauce. This is one recipe to which I like to add a touch of butter flavor.

2 tablespoons butter
2 tablespoons olive oil
1/4 cup all-purpose flour
1-1/3 cups fat-free milk or clam juice
1/3 cup low-fat evaporated milk
1/3 cup white wine
Dash nutmeg
1 teaspoon chopped fresh parsley
1 (6-oz.) can clams
Salt and pepper, to taste
2 cups cooked linguine
4 teaspoons grated Romano cheese

In a saucepan over medium heat, heat butter and oil and blend in flour. Cook, stirring, about 1 minute. Whisk in milk or clam juice, evaporated milk, and wine. Cook, stirring, until thickened. Add nutmeg, parsley, and clams with juice. Cover and simmer 5 minutes. Serve over hot linguine and sprinkle with Romano cheese. Makes 4 servings.

Each serving contains:

Cal	Prot	Carb	Fib	Tot. Fat	Sat. Fat	Chol	Sodium
370	17g	33g	1g	17g	7g	52mg	197mg

Shrimp, Beans, and Pasta

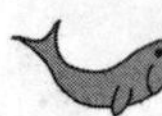

Enjoy this as a main dish for lunch or a light supper.

1/2 cup cooked or canned lima beans, drained
1 (6-oz.) can shrimp, drained
2 green onions, chopped
1 small zucchini, thinly sliced crosswise
2 tomatoes, chopped
6 pitted green olives, sliced
2 cups cooked mostaccioli or other pasta
1/3 cup Italian Dressing, page 107

If using canned beans, rinse and drain again. In a large mixing bowl, combine beans, shrimp, green onions, zucchini, tomatoes, and olives. Add hot cooked pasta. Toss all together with Italian Dressing. Serve at once, or cover and refrigerate 2 hours to thoroughly chill. Makes 6 servings.

Each serving contains:

Cal	Prot	Carb	Fib	Tot. Fat	Sat. Fat	Chol	Sodium
177	10g	17g	2g	8g	1g	49mg	147mg

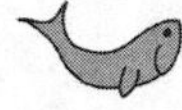

Spicy Beer-Marinated Shrimp Broil

Scallops, sea bass, or cod may be substituted for shrimp.

1 (12-oz.) can beer
1/4 teaspoon red chile pepper flakes
1/2 teaspoon dry mustard
1 tablespoon fresh lime juice
2 green onions, chopped
1/4 teaspoon sweet paprika
1/2 to 3/4 lb. raw shrimp, peeled, deveined

In a mixing bowl mix beer, chile flakes, mustard, lime, green onions, and paprika. Add shrimp and marinate in the refrigerator 3 to 4 hours.

Preheat broiler. Spray broiler pan with olive-oil cooking spray to prevent shrimp from sticking. Thread shrimp on 4 skewers. Broil at 450°F (230°C) or higher, 7 to 10 minutes until cooked. Turn at least once and brush with marinade if shrimp starts to dry out. Serve at once. Makes 4 servings.

Each serving contains:

Cal	Prot	Carb	Fib	Tot. Fat	Sat. Fat	Chol	Sodium
91	12g	3g	1g	1g	0g	86mg	88mg

Poultry

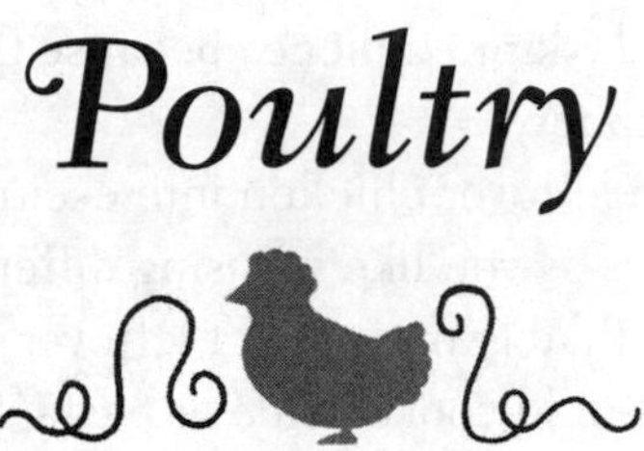

Chicken could easily be called a universal food; it is prepared in countless ways throughout the world. It's tender, tasty, inexpensive, always available, and lends itself to all methods of preparation.

Where applicable, I have given nutritional information for both white and dark meat. Those who are watching their fat and cholesterol intake can make a choice between white and dark meat. Choose whichever meets your needs.

When shopping for poultry, compare the per-pound pricing. Remember, poultry skin and bones account for 60 to 70 percent of the total weight. Sometimes boned, skinned chicken seems higher priced but can actually cost less for the edible portion.

The type of recipe you intend to make can be your guide as to which type of poultry you purchase. When making soups and salads, make the whole chicken your choice; if possible, buy a roaster. The mature bird has more flavor. I have used boneless, skinned chicken breasts often because of their lower fat content. However, if this is not your favorite piece, feel free to substitute other chicken parts. For instance, boneless thighs work just as well as the breasts do.

Marinating helps to tenderize and keep poultry moist. Marinades can be as simple as an Italian Dressing (page 107) barbecue sauce, or yogurt. Braising chicken is an easy and fast cooking method. Covering the pan during cooking also helps to seal in moisture. When grilling or barbecuing, turn pieces often to assure even cooking.

Because ovens differ so much, check for doneness when baking about 10 minutes before the time suggested in the recipe. Be careful not to overcook boned, skinned pieces because they can easily become tough and rubbery.

It is easy to turn leftover chicken into exciting new dishes. Personalize the recipes as you like by using different vegetables, fruits, or seasonings. Take two pieces of leftover chicken, remove the bones, and chop; then add cooked rice or pasta, fresh herbs, or nuts, and a bit of liquid—and you've created a casserole. Remember, you do not need a large portion of chicken to make a complete dish. For example, Barcelona Chicken Salad uses only 3/4 cup of cooked chicken and makes a wonderful entrée for six people.

Grilled Lemon Chicken

Whether you grill outside or broil inside, the results will be great.

1 lb. boneless, skinless chicken breasts
2 tablespoons fresh lemon juice
1 tablespoon grated lemon peel
1/2 teaspoon dried-leaf oregano
1/4 teaspoon sweet paprika
2 tablespoons olive or canola oil
1/4 cup chopped onion
1 clove garlic, chopped
1 tomato, chopped
3 oz. mozzarella cheese, thinly sliced
1 tablespoon chopped fresh basil
1 tablespoon chopped fresh parsley

Place chicken in a nonmetal bowl. Mix lemon juice, lemon peel, oregano, and paprika. Pour over chicken; turn pieces, cover, and refrigerate 1 hour.

Preheat grill or broiler. Heat oil in an 8-inch skillet over medium heat. Add onion and garlic and sauté until softened. Stir in tomato and set aside.

Grill or broil chicken until cooked through, about 20 minutes, turning as needed. Remove chicken from grill; place cheese and basil on top. Spoon tomato mixture over cheese. Return to grill or broiler; heat until cheese melts. Sprinkle with chopped parsley. Serve at once. Makes 4 servings.

Each serving with white meat contains:

Cal	Prot	Carb	Fib	Tot. Fat	Sat. Fat	Chol	Sodium
260	31g	4g	1g	13g	4g	82mg	156mg

Chicken Valencia

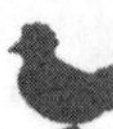

Prepare this simple combination of flavors that is reminiscent of Spain.

1 lb. chicken pieces, skinned, boned
1/2 teaspoon sweet paprika
2 teaspoons olive or canola oil
2 green onions, chopped
1/4 cup chopped fresh parsley
1 tomato, chopped
1/2 cup orange juice
1/4 cup raisins

Sprinkle chicken pieces with paprika, patting it in. Heat oil in a 10-inch skillet over medium heat. Add chicken and cook until brown, turning. Add remaining ingredients. Cover, reduce heat, and simmer until chicken is cooked through, 15 to 20 minutes. Turn chicken at least twice during cooking. Makes 4 servings.

Each serving with white meat contains:

Cal	Prot	Carb	Fib	Tot. Fat	Sat. Fat	Chol	Sodium
196	27g	13g	1g	4g	1g	66mg	83mg

Each serving with dark meat contains:

Cal	Prot	Carb	Fib	Tot. Fat	Sat. Fat	Chol	Sodium
340	20g	13g	1g	23g	6g	92mg	92mg

MARINATED CHICKEN AND GRAPES

Here is another way to combine chicken and fruit. This contains both fresh grapes and grape juice, both good sources of antioxidants.

Marinade:
- 2 tablespoons fresh lemon juice
- 2 tablespoons cider vinegar
- 1 tablespoon catsup
- 2 teaspoons olive or canola oil
- 1/4 cup white grape juice concentrate
- 1/4 teaspoon sweet paprika
- 1/2 teaspoon dry mustard
- 1 teaspoon dried-leaf basil
- 1/4 teaspoon onion powder

1 lb. boneless, skinless chicken breasts
2 teaspoons olive or canola oil
1 cup fresh green seedless grapes

Combine marinade ingredients in a medium nonmetal mixing bowl. Add chicken, cover, and refrigerate at least 2 hours.

In a 10-inch skillet, heat oil over medium heat. Remove chicken and pat dry, reserving marinade. Add chicken to skillet and brown lightly. Pour in marinade, cover, and simmer until chicken is cooked through, 15 to 20 minutes. Add grapes; cook until heated. Serve at once. Makes 4 servings.

Each serving with white meat contains:

Cal	Prot	Carb	Fib	Tot. Fat	Sat. Fat	Chol	Sodium
226	27g	14g	1g	6g	1g	66mg	122mg

Chicken Italiano

Serve over spinach fettuccine or your favorite pasta.

3/4 lb. chicken pieces, skinned, boned
2 green onions, chopped
1/2 cup low-sodium tomato sauce
2 tablespoons chopped dry-pack sun-dried tomatoes
1 tablespoon capers, rinsed
1/4 cup vermouth or white wine
2 tablespoons chopped fresh parsley
Salt and pepper to taste
2 cups cooked ziti or other pasta
1/4 cup grated Romano cheese

Spray a 10-inch skillet with olive-oil cooking spray. Heat over medium-low heat. Add chicken and brown on all sides; move pieces aside and sauté green onions. Remove skillet from heat and stir in tomato sauce, sun-dried tomatoes, capers, vermouth or wine, and parsley. Cover and simmer until chicken is cooked through, about 15 minutes. Season with salt and pepper. Serve over cooked pasta and sprinkle with cheese. Makes 4 servings.

Each serving with white meat contains:

Cal	Prot	Carb	Fib	Tot. Fat	Sat. Fat	Chol	Sodium
234	25g	21g	2g	3g	1g	56mg	311mg

Each serving with dark meat contains:

Cal	Prot	Carb	Fib	Tot. Fat	Sat. Fat	Chol	Sodium
342	20g	21g	2g	18g	6g	75mg	317mg

Chicken with Green Beans and Tomatoes

A colorful stovetop casserole; just serve with some crusty bread, and for dessert, fresh fruit.

2 teaspoons olive or canola oil
1 lb. chicken pieces, skinned, boned
1 garlic clove, minced
1/2 onion, chopped
1 (10-oz.) package frozen green beans
1 (16-oz.) can chopped tomatoes with juice
2 teaspoons fresh chopped parsley
1/2 teaspoon sweet paprika
Salt and pepper, to taste

Heat oil in a 12-inch skillet over medium heat. Add chicken and brown on all sides. Add garlic and onion and sauté until softened. Add green beans, tomatoes with juice, parsley, and paprika. Cover, reduce heat, and simmer until chicken is done, about 15 minutes. Season with salt and pepper. Makes 6 servings.

Each serving with white meat contains:

Cal	Prot	Carb	Fib	Tot. Fat	Sat. Fat	Chol	Sodium
131	19g	8g	2g	3g	0g	44mg	212mg

Each serving with dark meat contains:

Cal	Prot	Carb	Fib	Tot. Fat	Sat. Fat	Chol	Sodium
227	14g	8g	3g	16g	4g	61mg	218mg

Chicken, Rice, and Vegetable Casserole

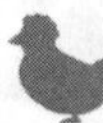

This dish can also be baked, but it will take longer to cook.

2 slices bacon, chopped
6 chicken thighs, skinned
1 cup long-grain white rice
1 small green or red bell pepper, chopped
1 small onion, chopped
1 cup chopped mushrooms (6 to 8 medium)
1 carrot, peeled, finely chopped
1-1/2 cups reduced-sodium canned chicken broth
1/2 cup dry white wine
Salt and pepper, to taste
2 teaspoons chopped fresh sage or 3/4 teaspoon dried-leaf
Sweet paprika
Chopped parsley

In a large skillet, cook bacon until crisp. Add chicken and brown lightly on all sides; remove to a plate. Add rice to skillet; cook, stirring, until rice begins to turn a light golden color. Add bell pepper, onion, mushrooms, carrot, broth, wine, salt, black pepper, and sage. Stir until well mixed. Arrange chicken thighs on top; sprinkle with paprika. Cover and simmer until chicken and rice are done, 35 to 40 minutes. Sprinkle with parsley. Makes 6 servings.

Each serving with dark meat contains:

Cal	Prot	Carb	Fib	Tot. Fat	Sat. Fat	Chol	Sodium
247	18g	29g	1g	5g	1g	59mg	344mg

BARCELONA CHICKEN SALAD

Create this beautiful main-dish salad with its combination of colors and flavors.

1/3 cup cooked green peas
2 tablespoons chopped pimiento
3/4 cup cubed cooked chicken
3 tablespoons orange juice
3 tablespoons olive or canola oil
1 green onion, chopped
1 tablespoon raisins
2 tablespoons chopped walnuts
Salt and pepper, to taste
Lettuce

In a large mixing bowl mix together peas, pimiento, and chicken; cover and refrigerate until chilled. In a cup, stir together orange juice, oil, green onion, raisins, and walnuts. Pour over chicken mixture. Toss gently. Season with salt and pepper. Line a serving dish with lettuce leaves; top with chicken mixture. Serve at once. Makes 6 servings.

Each serving with white meat contains:

Cal	Prot	Carb	Fib	Tot. Fat	Sat. Fat	Chol	Sodium
123	7g	4g	1g	9g	1g	15mg	71mg

Each serving with dark meat contains:

Cal	Prot	Carb	Fib	Tot. Fat	Sat. Fat	Chol	Sodium
130	6g	4g	1g	10g	1g	16mg	74mg

Sweet and Spicy Chicken with Peaches

Passion fruit juice gives this dish a taste of the tropics; guava juice could be substituted.

2 tablespoons olive or canola oil
1/2 onion, chopped
1 lb. chicken pieces, skinned, boned
1/2 teaspoon garlic powder
2 cups passion fruit juice
1/4 teaspoon red chile pepper flakes
1 tablespoon cornstarch
3 peaches, peeled, pitted, sliced

Heat oil in a 10-inch skillet over medium heat. Add onion and sauté until softened. Add chicken and brown lightly on all sides. Sprinkle with garlic powder. Add 1 cup of the passion fruit juice and chile flakes. Reduce heat, cover, and cook over medium heat about 15 minutes. Dissolve cornstarch in remaining passion fruit juice. Stir into skillet and cook, stirring, until slightly thickened. Add peach slices; cook about 5 minutes. Serve chicken topped with peaches and sauce. Makes 4 servings.

Each serving with white meat contains:

Cal	Prot	Carb	Fib	Tot. Fat	Sat. Fat	Chol	Sodium
294	27g	28g	2g	8g	1g	66mg	82mg

Each serving with dark meat contains:

Cal	Prot	Carb	Fib	Tot. Fat	Sat. Fat	Chol	Sodium
438	20g	28g	2g	28g	6g	92mg	91mg

Brandied Chicken and Apricots

Fresh ripe apricots are made even better with a hint of brandy and apricot preserves.

1/2 cup apricot preserves
1/4 cup boiling water
1 tablespoon brandy or brandy flavoring
1 teaspoon catsup
2 teaspoons fresh lemon or lime juice
1 teaspoon cornstarch
1 lb. chicken pieces
4 fresh apricots, quartered

Preheat oven to 375°F (190°C). Spray a baking dish large enough to hold chicken in a single layer with olive-oil cooking spray. Set aside. In a small bowl, combine apricot preserves, boiling water, brandy or brandy flavoring, catsup, lemon or lime juice, and cornstarch. Place chicken pieces in baking dish. Spoon sauce over. Bake uncovered, basting several times, about 30 minutes, until chicken is cooked through. Add apricots, spoon some of the sauce over, and bake 10 minutes. Makes 4 servings.

Each serving with white meat contains:

Cal	Prot	Carb	Fib	Tot. Fat	Sat. Fat	Chol	Sodium
253	57g	31g	1g	2g	0g	66mg	106mg

Each serving with dark meat contains:

Cal	Prot	Carb	Fib	Tot. Fat	Sat. Fat	Chol	Sodium
397	20g	31g	1g	21g	6g	92mg	115mg

Rice, Chicken, and Orange Casserole

Cold marinated asparagus, artichokes, or green beans make a good side dish.

1 cup long-grain white rice
1/2 cup reduced-sodium chicken broth
2 cups orange juice
2 tablespoons Zante currants
2 tablespoons chopped pistachios
3/4 lb. boneless, skinless chicken breasts
1/2 cup plain fat-free yogurt
1/2 teaspoon dried-leaf tarragon
Sweet paprika
1 orange, peeled, segmented

Preheat oven to 350˚F (180˚C). Spread rice evenly over bottom of a 5-1/2 quart Dutch oven. Combine chicken broth, orange juice, currants, and pistachios in a small mixing bowl. Pour over rice. Place chicken on top. Brush chicken with yogurt. Sprinkle with tarragon and paprika. Cover and bake about 30 minutes, until chicken is cooked through and rice is tender. Uncover, add orange segments, and bake about 15 minutes, or until chicken is browned. Makes 4 servings.

Each serving contains:

Cal	Prot	Carb	Fib	Tot. Fat	Sat. Fat	Chol	Sodium
391	27g	62g	3g	4g	1g	50mg	173mg

BAKED ROSEMARY CHICKEN

A crunchy baked coating of herbs and orange gives this dish special appeal.

2 lbs. chicken pieces, skinned
1/2 cup crushed corn cereal flakes
1 teaspoon crushed dried-leaf rosemary
1 1/2 teaspoons sweet paprika
1 1/2 teaspoons grated orange peel
1 teaspoon ground oregano
3/4 cup evaporated fat-free milk

Preheat oven to 375°F (190°C). Spray a baking sheet with olive-oil cooking spray. Remove all visible fat from chicken. Combine cereal, rosemary, paprika, orange peel, and oregano in a pie plate or small paper bag. Pour evaporated milk in another pie plate. Dip each chicken piece into milk mixture and then into cereal mixture. Place coated pieces on prepared baking sheet. Bake 30 to 40 minutes, or until chicken is browned and cooked through. Makes 4 servings.

Each serving with white meat contains:

Cal	Prot	Carb	Fib	Tot. Fat	Sat. Fat	Chol	Sodium
304	56g	9g	1g	3g	1g	133mg	235mg

Each serving with dark meat contains:

Cal	Prot	Carb	Fib	Tot. Fat	Sat. Fat	Chol	Sodium
592	42g	9g	1g	42g	12g	185mg	253mg

Meats

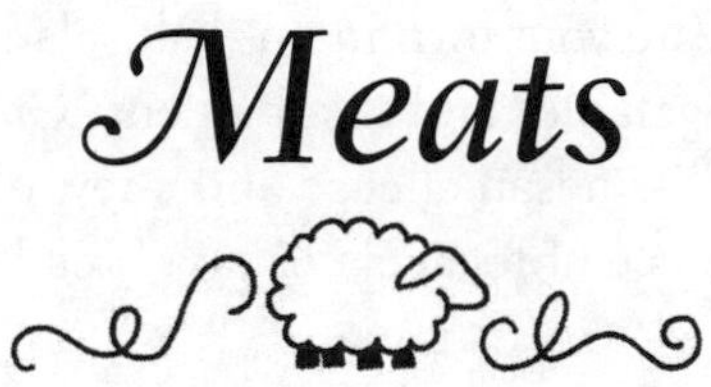

This chapter is smaller than others because the red meats are eaten in small amounts in this diet. They are used more to season a dish or are reserved for special occasions.

Lamb is probably the meat served most frequently, followed by veal. You'll find that the North African Lamb Kabobs are extra moist, tender, and flavorful when marinated in seasoned yogurt. (Although young goat meat is treasured by the Greeks for feast days, it is not available in our markets, so I have not included it.) Traditionally, braising beef as well as other meats has been a popular method of preparation. Long, slow cooking, often with wine, results in delicious, fork-tender meats.

I have included pork in my choice of recipes because it is a favorite, except for the Muslim countries, along the Mediterranean, particularly in Spain. Because of feeding methods, pork is not as fat as it was twenty years ago. Spinach-Stuffed Pork Roast is a delicious entrée for entertaining. You will also find hearty Meatballs Mozzarella, which is a great family dish.

Favorite embellishments once again reflect the products of these fertile lands. Lemon, capers, nuts, olives, and an assortment of cheeses, along with fresh herbs, add extra flavor to meat. To truly bring fresh flavor to meat dishes, do not be timid with fresh herbs. Although dried herbs are convenient, fresh herbs impart a special flavor. Many supermarkets now carry a variety of fresh herbs in the produce department. The next time you're shopping, buy some.

For an example of using meat as a minor ingredient, try this: Next time you have leftover roast or steak, slice it thinly and refrigerate. Then create your own main-dish salad by combining the chilled meat with vegetables and salad greens. Crown it with a sprinkling of feta or Parmesan cheese and a few olives on the side. Serve with a warm piece of focaccia or pita bread for a delicious meal.

Lamb Shanks, Vegetables, and Lentils

Serve with pasta, couscous, or rice. It's an ideal dish for your next party.

4 (1 lb.) lamb shanks
2 teaspoons olive oil
4 garlic cloves, sliced
1 onion, sliced
2 carrots, peeled, sliced
2 bay leaves
1 cup red wine
1 cup cooked lentils

Cut several slits in each lamb shank and brush with olive oil. Insert garlic slices in slits. In a large pot or Dutch oven, brown meat on all sides. Add onion, carrots, bay leaves, and wine. Cover and simmer until meat is tender, about 2 hours. Turn meat at least twice during cooking. Stir in lentils and cook until hot. Discard bay leaves and serve. Makes 4 servings.

Each serving contains:

Cal	Prot	Carb	Fib	Tot. Fat	Sat. Fat	Chol	Sodium
379	27g	18g	6g	18g	7g	82mg	99mg

North African Lamb Kabobs

Prepare kabobs and refrigerate in the yogurt marinade for up to 2 days before cooking.

- 1/2 cup plain fat-free yogurt
- 1/8 teaspoon ground cinnamon
- 1/8 teaspoon ground cloves
- 2 teaspoons chopped fresh parsley
- 1 tablespoon fresh lemon juice
- 1/2 teaspoon dried onion flakes
- 1/2 teaspoon fines herbes (a blend of dried chervil, chives, parsley, and tarragon)
- 1 lb. boneless leg of lamb, cut in 1-inch cubes, trimmed
- 18 cherry tomatoes
- 2 green bell peppers, cut in squares
- 1 onion, cut in 18 pieces
- 1 (10-oz.) package couscous, cooked

In a large mixing bowl, combine yogurt, cinnamon, cloves, parsley, lemon juice, onion flakes, and fines herbes. Add lamb and stir to coat all pieces. Cover and refrigerate 4 hours or overnight.

Preheat grill or broiler. Thread alternate pieces of lamb, tomatoes, bell pepper, and onion on metal skewers. Grill or broil, turning several times, until lamb is medium done, about 10 minutes, or to desired doneness. Serve with couscous. Makes 6 servings.

Each serving contains:

Cal	Prot	Carb	Fib	Tot. Fat	Sat. Fat	Chol	Sodium
360	30g	45g	4g	6g	2g	67mg	73mg

SPICY TURKISH GROUND LAMB

There are two ways to cook this mixture: One is to broil on skewers; the other is to shape in patties and pan fry.

3/4 lb. ground lean lamb
4 green onions, chopped
1/2 teaspoon garlic powder
1 tablespoon chopped fresh parsley
1/2 teaspoon sweet paprika
1/2 teaspoon dried-leaf oregano
1/2 teaspoon ground allspice
1/4 teaspoon ground cumin
1 egg white
Salt and pepper, to taste

Preheat broiler. In a bowl, thoroughly combine all ingredients. With wet hands, wrap mixture around 6 flat metal skewers, making a tapered cigar shape about 6 inches long. Or shape into patties. Place skewers or patties on a broiler rack. Cook 4 to 5 minutes per side, or to desired doneness. Makes 6 servings.

Each serving contains:

Cal	Prot	Carb	Fib	Tot. Fat	Sat. Fat	Chol	Sodium
83	12g	1g	1g	3g	1g	36mg	99mg

Pork Tenderloin

Herb flavors enhance the roast, but the cheese is unexpected.

1 (2-lb.) trimmed, boneless pork loin roast
1 teaspoon olive oil
3 garlic cloves, sliced
2 sprigs fresh rosemary or 2 teaspoons dried-leaf rosemary
4 fresh sage leaves or 1/2 teaspoon dried-leaf sage
1/2 cup crumbled feta or blue cheese

Preheat oven to 375°F (190°C). Place roast in a baking pan. Brush with oil. Cut 6 to 8 (1/2-inch-deep) slits in pork. Insert garlic into slits. Combine rosemary and sage; sprinkle over top. Press herbs lightly onto meat.

Roast about 2 hours, or until an instant-read thermometer registers between 160° to 170°F (70° to 75°C), depending on desired doneness. Remove to a serving platter. If using fresh herbs, remove them. Scatter cheese over all; cover and let stand for 5 minutes. Makes 6 servings.

Each serving contains:

Cal	Prot	Carb	Fib	Tot. Fat	Sat. Fat	Chol	Sodium
280	34g	1g	0g	14g	6g	103mg	206mg

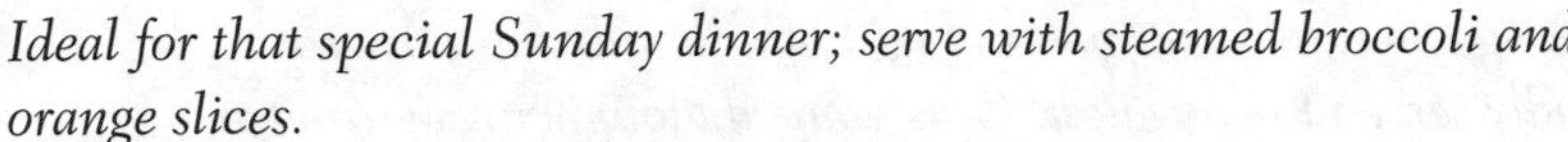

Spinach-Stuffed Pork Roast

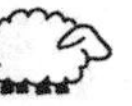

Ideal for that special Sunday dinner; serve with steamed broccoli and orange slices.

1 teaspoon dry mustard
1/2 teaspoon dried-leaf thyme
1/4 teaspoon grated nutmeg
1/2 teaspoon garlic powder
1 teaspoon grated orange peel
1 (1-lb.) trimmed pork tenderloin
1 (10-oz.) package frozen spinach, thawed, drained
2 tablespoons pine nuts
1 tablespoon chopped raisins
3 tablespoons low-sugar orange marmalade

Preheat oven to 350°F (175°C). In a cup, stir together mustard, thyme, nutmeg, garlic powder, and orange peel; set aside. Cut the meat in half lengthwise, cutting almost all the way through. Lay tenderloin open flat, sprinkle with 3/4 of herb mixture and pat into meat. Place spinach in a row down center of one tenderloin half. Sprinkle pine nuts and raisins on top. Lift other half of tenderloin over filling and secure by tying with string at 2-inch intervals, making a firm roll. Place on a baking rack; sprinkle remaining herbs on top, patting them in.

Roast about 40 minutes. Spread marmalade over top; roast 15 to 20 minutes more, or until an instant-read thermometer registers between 160° to 170°F (70° to 75°C), depending on desired doneness. Remove from oven, cover with foil, and let rest 10 to 15 minutes before slicing. Makes 4 servings.

Each serving contains:

Cal	Prot	Carb	Fib	Tot. Fat	Sat. Fat	Chol	Sodium
218	27g	13g	3g	7g	2g	74mg	114mg

Veal Stew

Although stew is sometimes thought of as family fare, this one can be proudly served to any guest. Crusty bread along with marinated artichokes would complement this dish.

1 tablespoon olive oil
3 tablespoons all-purpose flour
1 lb. boneless veal stew meat
1 onion, chopped
2 carrots, peeled, sliced
1 celery stalk, sliced
1 cup reduced-sodium canned chicken broth or water
2 potatoes, peeled, cubed
1/2 cup frozen green peas
1/4 cup plain fat-free yogurt
Salt and pepper, to taste

Heat oil in a large pan or Dutch oven over medium heat. Sprinkle 2 tablespoons of the flour over meat to coat and shake off excess. Brown meat in oil, turning. Add onion, carrots, celery, and broth or water. Cover and simmer about 20 minutes. Add potatoes and simmer until potatoes are cooked, about 35 minutes. Add peas. In a cup, blend remaining 1 tablespoon flour into yogurt. Stir yogurt mixture into juices to thicken sauce. Simmer, stirring, until thickened; do not boil. Season with salt and pepper. Makes 4 servings.

Each serving contains:

Cal	Prot	Carb	Fib	Tot. Fat	Sat. Fat	Chol	Sodium
282	27g	24g	3g	8g	2g	104mg	410mg

Veal with Lemon and Capers

Savor classic Mediterranean flavors—they're sure to please.

2 tablespoons olive oil
2 tablespoons all-purpose flour
1 lb. boneless veal scallops
1 egg, beaten
1 garlic clove, minced
2 tablespoons fresh lemon juice
1 tablespoon capers, drained
Chopped fresh parsley
Salt and pepper to taste

Heat oil in a large pan or Dutch oven over medium heat. Sprinkle flour over veal to coat and shake off excess. Dip into egg. Brown veal in oil, turning to cook on both sides. Add garlic and lemon juice. Simmer until veal is tender, about 5 minutes. Don't overcook or veal will be tough. Stir in capers and parsley. Season with salt and pepper. Makes 4 servings.

Each serving contains:

Cal	Prot	Carb	Fib	Tot. Fat	Sat. Fat	Chol	Sodium
297	32g	4g	0g	16g	4g	164mg	228mg

Beef Stew

Wine helps to tenderize the meat as well as impart delicious flavor.

1 tablespoon olive oil
2 tablespoons all-purpose flour
1 lb. boneless beef stew meat
2 garlic cloves, chopped
1 (10-oz.) package frozen petite whole onions
1 celery stalk, sliced
1 bay leaf
1 (15-oz.) can whole tomatoes
1-1/2 cups reduced-sodium canned beef broth or water
3/4 cup red wine
1 cup small whole button mushrooms
1 (15-oz.) can fava beans, drained
Salt and pepper to taste

Heat oil in a large pan or Dutch oven over medium heat. Sprinkle flour over meat to coat and shake off excess. Brown meat in oil, turning. Add garlic, onions, celery, bay leaf, tomatoes with juice, broth or water, and wine. Cover and simmer about 55 minutes until meat is fork tender. Add mushrooms and beans and cook 5 minutes. Season with salt and pepper. Makes 6 servings.

Each serving contains:

Cal	Prot	Carb	Fib	Tot. Fat	Sat. Fat	Chol	Sodium
391	27g	23g	5g	18g	6g	75mg	772mg

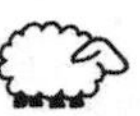

Meatballs Mozzarella

Tender meatballs have creamy cheese tucked inside. If you like, use half ground pork and half ground beef.

3 slices bread
1 lb. extra-lean ground beef
1 egg, beaten
1 garlic clove, minced
2 green onions, chopped
1/2 teaspoon dried-leaf thyme
2 tablespoons chopped fresh parsley
Salt and pepper, to taste
4 oz. mozzarella cheese, cut in 12 cubes
2 tablespoons olive oil
1 (8-oz.) can low-sodium tomato sauce
1/3 cup red wine

Soak bread in 1/2 cup water 3 to 4 minutes; squeeze out water and break up bread. Place in a bowl with beef, egg, garlic, green onions, thyme, and parsley. Thoroughly combine ingredients and season with salt and pepper. Form meatballs around cheese cubes, using about 1 tablespoon of meat mixture for each meatball.

Heat oil in a skillet or Dutch oven over medium heat. Brown meatballs on all sides. Add tomato sauce and wine. Reduce heat; cover and simmer until meatballs are cooked through, about 20 minutes. Makes 6 servings.

Each serving contains:

Cal	Prot	Carb	Fib	Tot. Fat	Sat. Fat	Chol	Sodium
351	21g	12g	1g	23g	9g	103mg	267mg

Italian Sausage with Lemon and Capers

I serve this flavorful sausage mixture as an omelet topping or a pita-bread filling or over cheese-filled manicotti.

1/2 lb. sweet or hot Italian sausage, sliced
2 tomatoes, seeded, chopped
2 tablespoons fresh lemon juice
1 tablespoon grated lemon peel
1 tablespoon capers, drained
1 tablespoon chopped fresh parsley
Salt and pepper, to taste

Heat a nonstick skillet over medium heat and brown sausage, turning frequently. Add tomatoes, lemon juice, lemon peel, and capers. Reduce heat; cover and cook until sausage is tender, about 10 minutes. If the mixture needs more liquid, add a little water. Stir in parsley and season with salt and pepper. Makes 4 servings.

Each serving contains:

Cal	Prot	Carb	Fib	Tot. Fat	Sat. Fat	Chol	Sodium
213	9g	4g	1g	18g	6g	43mg	557mg

Vegetables

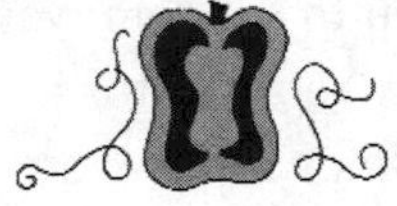

The wonderful climate of the Mediterranean region is ideal for growing vegetables. Commercial as well as home gardens provide flavorful, fresh produce year-round. Because of their abundance and variety, vegetables are used extensively in cooking. They add nutrition, color, texture, and flavor to meals. Meats, by comparison, are used sparingly.

An easy way to increase your consumption of vegetables is simply to take your favorite casserole or stir-fry recipe, reduce the meat by half, and double the amount of vegetables.

To help preserve flavor, color, and nutritional value of vegetables, cook them by steaming. You don't need special equipment, although steamers are handy. Simply place vegetables of uniform size in a vegetable-steamer basket or strainer or on a rack above a small amount of simmering water. Cover and cook until they are the desired tenderness, adding more water to the pot if needed. For a change of pace, season the water with a tablespoon of lemon juice or wine, or with herbs.

Another good way to prepare vegetables is to microwave them. Quick cooking in a microwave oven helps preserve color and texture. Be inventive—let my recipes serve as a guide to get you started in creative cooking.

Serve two or three vegetables at a meal rather than just one. You'll be amazed at how beautifully they enhance your meals. Make choices that lend contrast and color to your meal; for example, try pairing Sweet Potato Fritters with Squash, Tomato, Corn, Bean, and

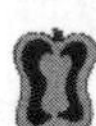

Feta Medley for a wonderful color combination and complementary flavors and textures. Or serve a chilled dish of Marinated Carrots with Green Olives along with a hot dish of Broccoli with Pine Nuts. The variety and combinations are almost unlimited; let creativity be your guide. You'll be delighted with the results.

To encourage children to eat their veggies, I keep a plastic bag of cut raw vegetables in the refrigerator for snacks. Offer these after school or between meals, knowing you are helping to establish good eating habits.

Cooking Oil Spray

If you like, make your own olive-oil cooking spray. Simply place 1 tablespoon olive oil in a small spray bottle and add 8 tablespoons water. Shake well before spraying.

Asparagus with Parmesan

This delicately flavored vegetable needs little embellishment.

2 lbs. fresh asparagus
2 teaspoons butter
1 teaspoon olive oil
1 tablespoon fresh lemon juice
1 tablespoon chopped fresh parsley
2 tablespoons grated Parmesan cheese

Trim off tough ends and peel asparagus stalks. If using very slim asparagus, peeling isn't necessary. Place in a steamer and cook 8 to 10 minutes. Heat butter and oil in a small skillet until butter melts, remove from heat, and stir in lemon juice and parsley. Place asparagus on a serving platter. Spoon lemon butter over top and sprinkle with cheese. Serve at once. Makes 4 or 5 servings.

Each serving contains:

Cal	Prot	Carb	Fib	Tot. Fat	Sat. Fat	Chol	Sodium
74	7g	7g	1g	4g	2g	6mg	51mg

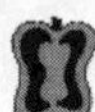

Beets in Fennel Sauce

This side dish is pretty served alongside a small amount of broiled meat or poultry.

1 (16-oz.) can sliced beets
2 teaspoons butter
1/4 cup chopped onion
1 teaspoon fennel seeds
1 tablespoon cornstarch
1 tablespoon cider vinegar
1 teaspoon grated lemon peel

Drain juice from beets, reserving 1/2 cup. In a saucepan over medium heat, melt butter. Add onion and fennel seeds and sauté until onion is softened. Add cornstarch to reserved beet juice and stir until dissolved. Add vinegar and lemon peel. Add to onion mixture and cook, stirring, until sauce thickens. Add beets and heat through. Makes 4 servings.

Each serving contains:

Cal	Prot	Carb	Fib	Tot. Fat	Sat. Fat	Chol	Sodium
65	1g	11g	2g	2g	1g	5mg	311mg

BROCCOLI WITH PINE NUTS

A spicy nut topping adds zest to this nutrient-packed vegetable.

3/4 lb. fresh broccoli or 1 (10-oz.) package frozen spears
2 teaspoons olive oil
1 green onion, chopped
2 garlic cloves, minced
3 tablespoons pine nuts
3 tablespoons raisins
1 tablespoon balsamic or red wine vinegar

If using fresh broccoli, trim ends and peel stalks. Place in a steamer basket; cover and steam about 10 minutes. For frozen broccoli, follow package instructions for cooking.

Heat oil in a small skillet over medium heat. Add green onion, garlic, pine nuts, and raisins and sauté until nuts are golden. Remove from heat and stir in vinegar. Place broccoli in a serving dish and spoon onion mixture over top. Makes 4 servings.

Each serving contains:

Cal	Prot	Carb	Fib	Tot. Fat	Sat. Fat	Chol	Sodium
105	4g	12g	2g	6g	1g	0mg	27mg

Cauliflower in Mustard Sauce

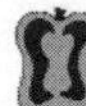

Mild mustard sauce adds color and new flavor to delicate cauliflower, which is high in beneficial antioxidants.

1 small head cauliflower or 1 (10-oz.) package frozen
1 teaspoon olive or canola oil
1 tablespoon butter
2 tablespoons chopped green onion
2 tablespoons all-purpose flour
1 cup milk
1 teaspoon Dijon mustard
1/2 cup shredded provolone cheese
Salt and pepper, to taste

If using fresh cauliflower, remove outer leaves from cauliflower, rinse, and separate into florets. In a saucepan, cover florets with water and boil until tender, about 8 minutes. If using frozen cauliflower, follow package directions for cooking. Remove cauliflower to serving dish, cover, and set aside.

In a small skillet, heat oil and butter over medium heat. Add onion and sauté until softened. Remove from heat and stir in flour. Return to heat and slowly stir in milk. Cook, stirring, until thickened. Stir in mustard and cheese. Cook, stirring, until cheese is blended in sauce. Season with salt and pepper. Pour sauce over cauliflower. Serve at once. Makes 4 servings.

Each serving contains:

Cal	Prot	Carb	Fib	Tot. Fat	Sat. Fat	Chol	Sodium
184	10g	14g	3g	11g	6g	27mg	324mg

Brussels Sprouts with Currants and Walnuts

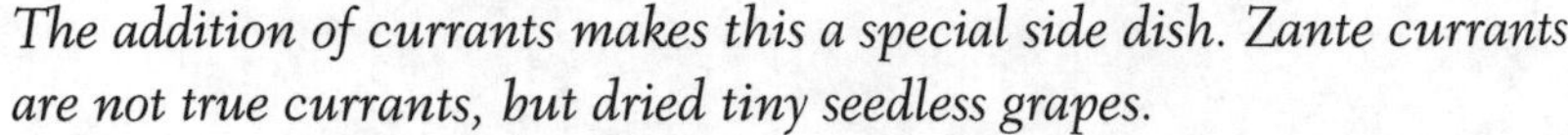

The addition of currants makes this a special side dish. Zante currants are not true currants, but dried tiny seedless grapes.

1-1/4 cups reduced-sodium canned chicken broth
1/4 onion, sliced
2 (16-oz.) packages frozen Brussels sprouts
2 strips bacon, cooked, crumbled
2 tablespoons balsamic vinegar
1/4 cup Zante currants
1/4 cup chopped walnuts
Salt and pepper, to taste

Combine chicken broth, onion, and Brussels sprouts in a saucepan. Cook until sprouts are tender, about 15 minutes. Remove to a serving bowl. Toss with bacon, vinegar, currants, and walnuts. Season with salt and pepper. Serve at once. Makes 6 servings.

Each serving contains:

Cal	Prot	Carb	Fib	Tot. Fat	Sat. Fat	Chol	Sodium
115	6g	15g	4g	5g	1g	2mg	256mg

Braised Red Cabbage

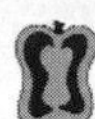

A good and hearty side dish, full of wonderful flavor—and beneficial antioxidants.

1 tablespoon olive or canola oil
1 onion, chopped
1 lb. red cabbage, cored, shredded
2 apples, peeled, cored, sliced
1 teaspoon sugar
1/2 cup unsalted tomato juice
1/4 teaspoon ground cloves
1/4 teaspoon grated nutmeg
1/4 cup chopped almonds
1/2 cup red wine

Heat oil in a large sauté pan over medium heat. Add onion and sauté until softened. Stir in cabbage and apples; stir-fry until cabbage wilts. Add sugar, tomato juice, cloves, nutmeg, and almonds. Cover and simmer about 10 minutes. Stir in wine and cook about 5 minutes longer. Serve hot. Makes 6 servings.

Each serving contains:

Cal	Prot	Carb	Fib	Tot. Fat	Sat. Fat	Chol	Sodium
125	3g	16g	3g	6g	1g	0mg	13mg

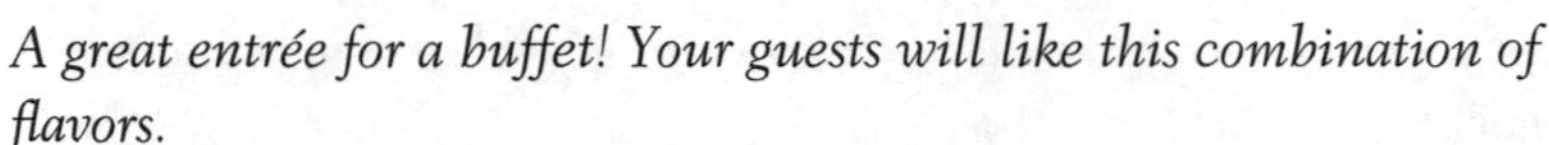

Baked Eggplant and Rice with Mushroom Sauce

A great entrée for a buffet! Your guests will like this combination of flavors.

1 (1-lb.) eggplant, cut lengthwise in 8 slices
Salt
1 tablespoon plus 1 teaspoon olive oil
2 green onions, chopped
2 garlic cloves, minced
4 teaspoons cornstarch
1/2 cup orange juice
1/2 cup reduced-sodium canned chicken broth
1/2 cup fat-free milk
1/2 teaspoon dried-leaf sage
1 teaspoon grated orange peel
1 cup sliced fresh mushrooms
2 cups cooked rice
2 tomatoes

Preheat oven to 350°F (175°C). Sprinkle eggplant lightly with salt; set aside 10 minutes. Pat with paper towel to remove excess moisture. Brush slices with the 1 teaspoon oil and brown both sides in a large skillet over medium heat. In a fry pan, heat the 1 tablespoon oil over medium heat. Add green onions and garlic and sauté until softened. Dissolve cornstarch in orange juice and chicken broth; stir into onion and garlic. Add milk, sage, and orange peel. Simmer, stirring, until mixture has thickened. Stir in mushrooms. Spoon rice into a 13 x 9-inch baking dish. Place eggplant slices in one layer over rice. Cut each tomato in 4 slices and place on top of eggplant. Pour mushroom sauce over all. Cover and bake about 25 minutes. Makes 8 servings.

Each serving contains:

Cal	Prot	Carb	Fib	Tot. Fat	Sat. Fat	Chol	Sodium
116	3g	21g	2g	3g	1g	2mg	98mg

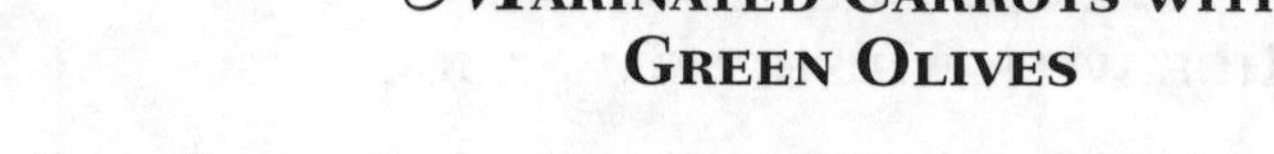

Marinated Carrots with Green Olives

For a change of pace, prepare cauliflower or green beans in the same manner.

- 2 lbs. fresh carrots, peeled and sliced crosswise, or 2 (10-oz.) packages frozen sliced carrots
- 2 tablespoons chopped fresh parsley
- 3 tablespoons chopped pimiento-stuffed olives
- 1/2 cup Italian Dressing, page 107

In a saucepan, cook fresh carrots in water to cover until crisp-tender, 10 to 12 minutes; drain. If using frozen carrots, cook according to package directions; drain. Combine carrots, parsley, and olives in a shallow bowl. Pour Italian Dressing over carrot mixture. Cover and refrigerate at least 2 hours. Stir twice while chilling. Makes 6 servings.

Each serving contains:

Cal	Prot	Carb	Fib	Tot. Fat	Sat. Fat	Chol	Sodium
151	2g	16g	5g	10g	1g	0mg	123mg

Leeks with Tarragon Sauce

This elegant member of the onion family deserves more attention from cooks. Leeks, which look like very large scallions, have a mild flavor.

4 leeks
1-1/2 cups reduced-sodium canned chicken broth
1 teaspoon dried-leaf tarragon
1/4 cup vermouth or fresh lemon juice
1/2 cup chopped red bell pepper
2 tablespoons cornstarch
1/4 cup fat-free milk
1 tablespoon chopped chives
Salt and pepper, to taste

Trim dark green portions and roots from leeks. Cut in half lengthwise; thoroughly rinse to remove dirt. In a large sauté pan over medium heat, bring chicken broth to a boil. Add leeks; cover and simmer until tender, 7 to 10 minutes. Remove leeks to a serving dish; cover and keep warm. Add tarragon, vermouth or lemon juice, and bell pepper to broth. Dissolve cornstarch in milk. Stir into broth. Cook, stirring, until thickened. Add chives. Season with salt and pepper. Pour sauce over leeks. Serve at once. Makes 4 servings.

Each serving contains:

Cal	Prot	Carb	Fib	Tot. Fat	Sat. Fat	Chol	Sodium
114	4g	20g	2g	1g	0g	0mg	393mg

Sweet Potato Fritters

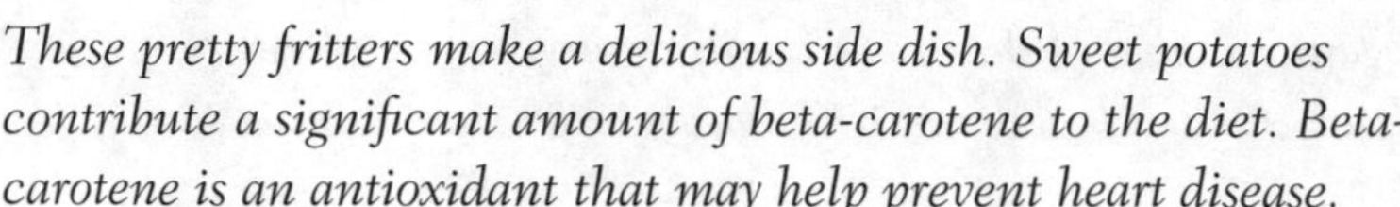

These pretty fritters make a delicious side dish. Sweet potatoes contribute a significant amount of beta-carotene to the diet. Beta-carotene is an antioxidant that may help prevent heart disease.

1 (8-oz.) sweet potato, peeled, shredded
1 carrot, peeled, shredded
1 tablespoon minced onion
2 eggs or 1/2 cup egg substitute
1/4 cup all-purpose flour
3 tablespoons orange juice
1 tablespoon grated orange peel
2 tablespoons chopped fresh parsley
Salt and pepper, to taste
1 to 2 tablespoons olive or canola oil

In a medium bowl, thoroughly combine all ingredients except oil. In a 12-inch sauté pan, heat oil over medium heat. For each fritter, carefully spoon about 2 tablespoons of the sweet-potato mixture into pan. Press lightly to form fritters. When edges begin to brown, turn; then lightly press again and cook other side until browned. Place on paper towels, cover to keep warm, and cook remaining sweet potato mixture. Makes 10 to 12 fritters.

Each fritter contains:

Cal	Prot	Carb	Fib	Tot. Fat	Sat. Fat	Chol	Sodium
68	2g	10g	1g	2g	1g	43mg	48mg

BELL PEPPERS FLORENTINE

Make a double amount and freeze half before baking. For a colorful presentation, use a combination of red, yellow, and orange bell peppers.

1 (10-oz.) package frozen chopped spinach
1/2 lb. ground beef
1 garlic clove, minced
1 small onion, minced
1/4 teaspoon dried-leaf basil
1/4 teaspoon dried-leaf oregano
2 tablespoons raisins
1/2 cup cooked rice
2 tablespoons unsalted tomato paste
1 egg white, slightly beaten
4 green bell peppers, seeded, stem ends removed
2 teaspoons chopped pimiento
2 teaspoons chopped parsley

Preheat oven to 375°F (190°C). Spray a 10 X 8-inch baking dish with olive-oil cooking spray. Thaw spinach and drain, squeezing out as much liquid as possible. Set aside.

Spray a small skillet with olive-oil cooking spray. Add beef, garlic, and onion. Cook until beef is browned, stirring to break up; drain off excess fat.

In a mixing bowl combine spinach, beef mixture, basil, oregano, raisins, rice, tomato paste, and egg white. Fill peppers with mixture and top with pimiento and parsley. Place in prepared baking dish. Bake about 30 minutes, or until tops are browned. Makes 4 servings.

Each serving contains:

Cal	Prot	Carb	Fib	Tot. Fat	Sat. Fat	Chol	Sodium
236	17g	23g	5g	9g	3g	90mg	103mg

Baked Herbed Potato Wedges

So simple, so good! Vary the seed-and-herb topping to suit your taste.

2 large baking potatoes, unpeeled
2 tablespoons olive oil
1/4 teaspoon cumin seeds
1 teaspoon dried-leaf oregano
1 teaspoon dried-leaf thyme
Salt and pepper, to taste

Preheat oven to 425°F (220°C). Scrub potatoes; pat dry. Cut potatoes lengthwise into eighths. Brush with oil and place in a baking dish. Sprinkle with cumin seeds, oregano, and thyme. Bake about 35 minutes, or until potatoes are tender. Season with salt and pepper. Makes 4 servings.

Each serving contains:

Cal	Prot	Carb	Fib	Tot. Fat	Sat. Fat	Chol	Sodium
162	2g	24g	3g	7g	1g	0mg	80mg

Squash, Tomato, Corn, Bean, and Feta Medley

Feta cheese adds extra flavor to a colorful medley of vegetables that's sure to please almost everyone.

2 crookneck squash (1 lb.), thinly sliced
2 pattypan squash (1 lb.), thinly sliced
2 tomatoes, seeded, chopped
1 (12-oz.) can cream-style corn
3 green onions, chopped
1 (15-oz.) can cannellini (white kidney) beans, drained, rinsed
1/2 cup crumbled feta cheese
2 teaspoons chopped fresh mint
1 teaspoon dried-leaf oregano
1 teaspoon dried-leaf marjoram
Salt and pepper, to taste

Preheat oven to 350°F (175°C). Spray a 2-quart casserole with olive-oil cooking spray. Combine squash, tomatoes, corn, green onions, and beans in casserole. Cover and bake 30 minutes. Sprinkle cheese over vegetables. Scatter mint, oregano, and marjoram on top of cheese. Bake uncovered 10 to 12 minutes. Season with salt and pepper. Makes 8 servings.

Each serving contains:

Cal	Prot	Carb	Fib	Tot. Fat	Sat. Fat	Chol	Sodium
137	6g	24g	6g	3g	1g	8mg	410mg

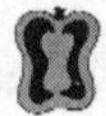

Zucchini, Mushrooms, and Onion with Sage

Yellow and green zucchini taste the same; mixing the colors in this dish creates added visual interest.

- 2 tablespoons olive or canola oil
- 1 cup zucchini slices
- 1 cup onion slices
- 1 cup sliced fresh mushrooms
- 2 tablespoons cornstarch
- 2/3 cup reduced-sodium canned chicken broth
- 1/4 cup dry sherry
- 1 tablespoon chopped fresh sage leaves or 1 teaspoon dried-leaf
- 1/2 teaspoon sweet paprika
- 3 tablespoons dry bread crumbs
- 2 tablespoons grated Parmesan cheese

Preheat oven to 350°F (175°C). Spray a 1-quart baking dish with olive-oil cooking spray. Heat oil in a large fry pan over medium heat. Add zucchini and onion and sauté until softened. Stir in mushrooms. Transfer zucchini mixture to baking dish. In a cup, combine cornstarch with chicken broth, sherry, sage, and paprika. Pour over zucchini. Combine bread crumbs and Parmesan cheese. Sprinkle on top. Bake uncovered about 25 minutes, or until hot and bubbly. Makes 4 to 6 servings.

Each serving contains:

Cal	Prot	Carb	Fib	Tot. Fat	Sat. Fat	Chol	Sodium
152	4g	13g	2g	8g	1g	2mg	236mg

Baked Mixed Vegetables

When fixing a roast, put this dish in the oven during the last 20 minutes of baking.

2 (16-oz.) packages frozen mixed vegetables
1 cup reduced-sodium canned beef broth
1/2 teaspoon dried-leaf basil
1/2 teaspoon dried-leaf tarragon
2 teaspoons chopped fresh parsley

Preheat oven to 350˚F (175˚C). Spray a 2-quart baking dish with olive-oil spray. Combine all ingredients in prepared baking dish. Cook covered about 25 minutes, stirring occasionally. Serve hot or cold. Makes 6 servings.

Each serving contains:

Cal	Prot	Carb	Fib	Tot. Fat	Sat. Fat	Chol	Sodium
100	6g	21g	6g	1g	0g	0mg	202mg

Potatoes, Onions, Carrots, and Peas

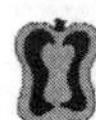

A colorful side dish, full of vegetables, to serve with Macaroni Frittata, page 125.

1/2 lb. small whole onions, peeled
1 lb. small new potatoes, cubed
3 carrots, peeled, thinly sliced into rounds
1 cup reduced-sodium canned chicken broth
1 tablespoon chopped fresh parsley
Salt and pepper, to taste
1 cup frozen green peas

Spray a saucepan with olive-oil cooking spray. Add onions and cook over medium-low heat until lightly browned. Add all remaining ingredients except peas; bring to a boil. Reduce heat. Cover and simmer until vegetables are tender, 20 to 30 minutes. Add peas and cook 5 minutes longer. Makes 6 servings.

Each serving contains:

Cal	Prot	Carb	Fib	Tot. Fat	Sat. Fat	Chol	Sodium
95	4g	19g	4g	1g	0g	0mg	195mg

Breads

Most of us begin the day with bread or cereal and juice or coffee before going off to work. Make that simple beginning memorable by serving Anise Bread. A delightful choice for toast, its fragrance will entice even the sleepiest in your household to the breakfast table. Honey–Poppy Seed Bread is an excellent all-purpose bread, delicious plain or toasted for breakfast and also great for sandwiches later in the day.

Traditional French Bread is probably the most popular bread of all. The recipe on page 206 makes two loaves, one for today and one for tomorrow. Or if you like, make one loaf and form the remaining dough into rolls. Making French Bread and other yeast breads can be time-consuming, but the rewards in terms of taste and nutrition make the effort worthwhile.

For a more substantial bread, try Olive Focaccia. I personally like this for lunch or dinner, but others prefer it warmed for breakfast—enjoy it either way. The beauty of focaccia is that it can be changed easily to suit your personal flavor preferences. Feel free to substitute other ingredients if olives are not your favorite topping. You might experiment with onions, capers, chopped sun-dried tomatoes, or a liberal sprinkling of fresh herbs and freshly ground black pepper.

Pizza, anyone? Of course! Everyone likes pizza. Once you have made your own Pizza Dough, you will no longer be satisfied with the store-bought variety. The possibilities for pizza toppings are almost endless. I've included one to get you started. In Italy, the basic cheese-and-tomato pie is called Pizza Margarita. Simply add your favorite herbs and enjoy!

ANISE BREAD

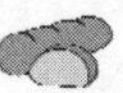

Toast slices for the best-tasting sandwiches you've ever eaten.

1/4 cup olive oil
1 tablespoon brown sugar
1 cup warm milk (105–115°F; 40–45°C)
1/2 teaspoon salt
1 teaspoon anise seeds
1/2 teaspoon anise flavoring
1 (1/4-oz.) package active dry yeast (about 1 tablespoon)
1 egg, beaten
3-1/2 cups all-purpose flour

In a mixer bowl, combine oil, brown sugar, milk, salt, anise seeds, anise flavoring, and yeast. Let stand until foamy, about 5 minutes. With mixer running, blend in egg and 2 cups of the flour. Add as much more flour as needed to make a soft dough. Turn dough out on a lightly floured surface and knead in remaining flour.

Place dough in a lightly oiled bowl, cover, and let rise in a warm, draft-free place until double in bulk, about 1-1/2 hours. Turn dough out, punch down, and form into loaf shape. Place in a greased 9 X 5-inch loaf pan. Cover and let rise until almost double in bulk, about 30 minutes.

Preheat oven to 375°F (190°C). Bake 35 to 40 minutes, or until golden brown and loaf sounds hollow when tapped on bottom. Remove from pan and cool. Cut into 16 slices. Makes 1 loaf.

Each slice contains:

Cal	Prot	Carb	Fib	Tot. Fat	Sat. Fat	Chol	Sodium
148	4g	23g	1g	5g	1g	15mg	85mg

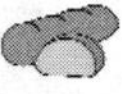

HONEY–POPPY SEED BREAD

A good all-purpose loaf the whole family will enjoy. You'll love the flavor.

1/3 cup honey
2 cups hot water
2 tablespoons butter
1 tablespoon poppy seeds
1 cup rolled oats
1 (1/4-oz.) package active dry yeast (about 1 tablespoon)
1/4 cup warm water (105–115°F; 40–45°C)
4-1/2 to 5 cups all-purpose flour

In a mixer bowl, stir together honey, hot water, butter or margarine, and poppy seeds. Stir in oats. Set aside for 15 to 20 minutes. In a cup, stir yeast in warm water; let stand until foamy, 5 minutes; add to oat mixture. Use a dough hook to beat in about 4 cups of the flour. Mix thoroughly. Turn out on a lightly floured board. Knead, adding more flour as necessary, to make a smooth satiny dough. Place dough in a large oiled bowl, turning dough to coat all sides. Cover; let rise in a warm, draft-free place about 1-1/2 hours, until doubled in bulk.

Punch down dough; cover and let dough rest 5 minutes. Shape into 2 loaves. Place in 2 greased 9 X 5-inch pans. Let rise until almost doubled in bulk, about 30 minutes.

Preheat oven to 375°F (190°C). Bake about 50 minutes, or until loaves sound hollow when tapped on bottoms. Remove from pan and cool. Cut each loaf into 16 slices. Makes 2 loaves.

Each slice contains:

Cal	Prot	Carb	Fib	Tot. Fat	Sat. Fat	Chol	Sodium
93	2g	18g	1g	1g	1g	2mg	1mg

Pizza Dough

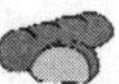

Top with sausage, meat, cheese or Onion-Tomato Topping, page 205.

1 (1/4-oz.) package active dry yeast (about 1 tablespoon)
1 cup warm water (105–115°F; 40–45°C)
2 teaspoons olive oil
1/2 teaspoon salt
2-1/2 to 3 cups all-purpose flour

In a mixer bowl, dissolve yeast in warm water; let stand until foamy, about 5 minutes. Add oil, salt, and 2 cups of the flour. Beat until thoroughly combined, making a soft dough. Turn dough out onto a floured surface. Knead in enough flour to make a stiff dough. Spray a bowl with olive-oil cooking spray. Place dough in bowl, cover, and let rise in a warm, draft-free place until doubled in bulk.

Preheat oven to 450°F (230°C). Punch down dough; cut in half and roll out to fit 2 (12-inch) pizza pans. Top with favorite topping. Bake 15 to 20 minutes until browned. Makes 2 (12-inch) pizzas.

Each 2-inch slice without topping contains:

Cal	Prot	Carb	Fib	Tot. Fat	Sat. Fat	Chol	Sodium
52	1g	10g	0g	1g	0g	0mg	49mg

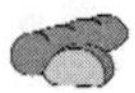

Onion-Tomato Topping

For a quick lunch, try this topping on toasted French bread.

1 tablespoon olive oil
2 onions, thinly sliced into rings
3 tomatoes, thinly sliced
1/4 cup sliced black olives
2 cups (8 oz.) shredded mozzarella cheese
Dried-leaf basil, to taste
Dried-leaf oregano, to taste
Pepper, to taste

In a skillet, heat olive oil over medium heat. Add onions and sauté until softened. Arrange onions on top of pizza dough. Top with sliced tomatoes, olives, and cheese. Sprinkle with basil, oregano, and pepper. Makes enough topping for 2 (12-inch) pizzas.

Topping for each 2-inch slice contains:

Cal	Prot	Carb	Fib	Tot. Fat	Sat. Fat	Chol	Sodium
43	2g	2g	0g	3g	1g	7mg	55mg

French Bread

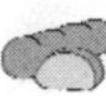

Variations of this type of bread are found in many countries other than France.

2-1/4 cups warm water (105–115°F; 40–45°C)
1 (1/4-oz.) package active dry yeast (about 1 tablespoon)
1 teaspoon sugar (optional)
6 to 6-1/2 cups all-purpose or bread flour
1 teaspoon salt
2 tablespoons cornmeal
Glaze:
1 egg white
1 tablespoon water

Pour water into a large mixer bowl; stir in yeast and sugar, if using. Let stand until yeast is foamy, about 5 minutes. Beat in 2 cups of the flour and the salt and mix well. Add enough of the remaining flour to make a moderately stiff and manageable dough. Turn dough out onto a lightly floured board; knead by hand 5 to 7 minutes. Dough should be smooth and elastic. Lightly oil a large bowl. Place dough in bowl; turn to coat all sides. Cover top of bowl with plastic wrap or a damp cloth. Place in a warm, draft-free area. Let dough rise until doubled in bulk, about 2 hours, depending on room temperature. Punch dough down and turn in bowl, cover again, and let rise.

Grease a baking sheet and sprinkle with cornmeal. Set aside. Turn dough out onto a floured surface. Punch down, cover, and let rest about 5 minutes. Shape dough into 2 long loaves and place on prepared baking sheet. Cover and let rise until doubled, about 1 hour.

Preheat oven to 425°F (220°C). With a sharp knife or razor, cut several slashes in tops of bread. For glaze, beat egg white and water together in a small bowl. Lightly brush tops with glaze. Bake 10 minutes. For a crisper crust, brush tops with glaze again. Bake another 10 minutes and repeat brushing with glaze. Bake another 20 minutes, until browned and loaves sound hollow when tapped on bottoms. Total baking time is about 40 minutes. Cool and cut each loaf into 16 slices. Makes 2 loaves.

Each slice contains:

Cal	Prot	Carb	Fib	Tot. Fat	Sat. Fat	Chol	Sodium
88	3g	18g	1g	0g	0g	0mg	75mg

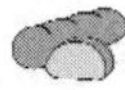

Olive Focaccia

Versatile bread that can accompany a meal or be used for sandwiches.

1 (1/4-oz.) package active dry yeast (about 1 tablespoon)
3/4 cup warm water (105–115°F; 40–45°C)
1/2 teaspoon salt
1-1/2 cups all-purpose flour
1-1/4 cups whole-wheat flour
4 tablespoons olive oil
2 tablespoons chopped fresh basil
2 tablespoons cornmeal
1/4 cup chopped Kalamata olives
1/4 cup grated Romano cheese

In a mixer bowl, dissolve yeast in warm water. Let stand until yeast is foamy. Add salt, all-purpose flour, and 1/2 cup whole-wheat flour. Beat until thoroughly combined, making a soft dough. Beat in 3 tablespoons of the olive oil and basil. Turn dough out onto a floured surface. Knead about 5 minutes, adding flour as necessary to make a moderately stiff dough. Brush a bowl with olive oil. Place dough in bowl, turn dough to coat all sides. Cover and let rise in a warm, draft-free area until doubled in bulk, about 1 hour.

Punch down dough, let rest for 5 minutes. Oil a 13 X 9-inch baking pan; sprinkle with cornmeal. Pat dough into pan. With fingertips, make 1/2-inch deep dimples over the surface. Brush with remaining 1 tablespoon olive oil and scatter with olives, pressing them into dough. Sprinkle with cheese.

Preheat oven to 425°F (220°C). Cover and let rise 15 minutes.

Bake 15 to 20 minutes, until lightly browned. Cut into serving pieces. Serve warm or cooled. Makes 8 to 10 servings.

Each serving contains:

Cal	Prot	Carb	Fib	Tot. Fat	Sat. Fat	Chol	Sodium
251	7g	33g	3g	10g	2g	3mg	156mg

Sweet Fruit Bread

Dried and candied fruits can be used in a variety of breads. This version is especially nice toasted.

1/2 cup sugar
1/4 cup butter
1 egg
1 teaspoon grated lemon peel
1 teaspoon anise extract
3 cups all-purpose flour
2 teaspoons baking powder
1/2 teaspoon salt
1 cup fat-free milk
3/4 cup mixed candied fruits
1/4 cup chopped walnuts

Preheat oven to 325°F (165°C). Butter 2 (9 X 5-inch) loaf pans. In a mixer bowl, cream together sugar and butter. Beat in egg, lemon peel, and anise extract. Combine flour, baking powder, and salt. Alternately add dry ingredients and milk, beating after each addition. Beat until thoroughly combined. Stir in fruits and nuts.

Spoon into prepared pans. Bake about 45 minutes, or until wooden pick inserted in centers comes out clean. Cool in pan 10 minutes. Turn out on cooling rack. Cut each loaf into 16 slices. Makes 2 loaves.

Each slice contains:

Cal	Prot	Carb	Fib	Tot. Fat	Sat. Fat	Chol	Sodium
96	2g	16g	0g	3g	1g	12mg	60mg

Desserts

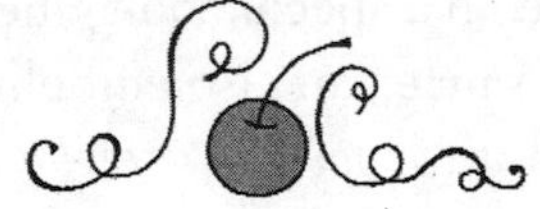

Naturally sweet, fresh fruits dominate this chapter. In Mediterranean homes, dessert is a routine after-dinner feature. When dessert is offered, it's usually fruit-based. We would all benefit from reducing the amounts of sweets we consume after dinner. Unfortunately, we have acquired the habit of expecting a dessert, and it's difficult to break.

We can still look forward to that final touch of a lovely meal without feeling guilty if we concentrate on keeping it light in calories and fat. The answer is to serve light fruit desserts, which offer fresh flavors and bright, enticing colors. Similar to a palate cleanser, a less rich dessert doesn't leave you feeling uncomfortable. It is truly a pleasant way to end a delightful dinner. Reserve richer desserts for special occasions and holidays as the people of the Mediterranean do.

It seems increasingly difficult to buy tree-ripened fruit, bursting with flavor, so plan to purchase produce in ample time to allow for ripening. As a rule, ripe fruit has a pleasant aroma; in general, no aroma means no flavor.

Some desserts in this chapter require a certain amount of preparation time, while others can be made picture-perfect in minutes. For those times when you crave the occasional high-calorie treat after a light meal, you'll find Oranges and Raspberries with Mascarpone, a beautiful dish that takes just minutes to prepare. Simple puddings such as Café au Lait Pudding are fine alone or can be accompanied with Almond Cookies. This ideal combination pairs a velvety pudding with a crunchy cookie for a delightful contrast in texture and flavor.

Cool, palate-pleasing Lemon Gelato is everyone's favorite on a warm summer day. It's tangy and refreshing without being too sweet. But don't wait until summer to enjoy it—I like it any time of the year.

Apple Fritters take on a special look when lightly topped with a Blackberry Sauce. This sauce can also embellish other fresh fruits or ice cream, so don't limit it to just one use!

Hazelnut Biscotti will delight all who are lucky enough to try these crunchy cookies. Store them in an airtight container to preserve their texture. The best way to enjoy them is by dunking them into coffee or wine to soften them a bit.

Orange-Almond Crêpes

Light crêpes are filled with fresh fruit, almonds, and ricotta cheese.

1 cup all-purpose flour
3 eggs
1-1/2 cups milk
1 tablespoon extra-light olive oil
1 teaspoon orange or vanilla extract
Olive oil for frying
Ricotta, Orange, and Almond Filling, page 212
Powdered sugar (optional)

In a food processor or blender, combine flour, eggs, milk, oil, and extract. Process until combined. Set aside for 30 minutes.

Lightly brush a crêpe pan or a 6- to 7-inch skillet with oil. For each crêpe, pour about 2 tablespoons batter into heated pan, and immediately tilt pan so batter covers the bottom. Cook until surface looks dry and edges are lacy and brown. At this point, you can flip the crêpe onto a warm plate, because only one side needs to be cooked. Or if you like the crêpe a little more colored, flip it over in pan and cook other side for a few seconds; do not overcook.

To fill crêpes, place a heaping tablespoon of filling in the center of the crêpe and spread within an inch of the edge. Fold in half or roll up. Dust with sifted powdered sugar, if desired. Makes about 12 crêpes.

Each non-filled crêpe contains:

Cal	Prot	Carb	Fib	Tot. Fat	Sat. Fat	Chol	Sodium
91	4g	10g	0g	4g	2g	60mg	31mg

Each filled crêpe contains:

Cal	Prot	Carb	Fib	Tot. Fat	Sat. Fat	Chol	Sodium
201	10g	17g	1g	11g	6g	81mg	71mg

RICOTTA, ORANGE, AND ALMOND FILLING

You may also use the filling as a topping for fresh fruits.

2 cups ricotta or small-curd cottage cheese
1/2 cup plain fat-free yogurt or fat-free dairy sour cream
3 to 4 tablespoons sugar
2 tablespoons grated orange peel
1 orange, peeled and chopped
1/4 cup blanched almonds, chopped

In a bowl, thoroughly combine ricotta or cottage cheese, yogurt or sour cream, and sugar. Stir in remaining ingredients.

Makes enough filling for 12 crêpes (about 1 cup).

1/12 of filling contains:

Cal	Prot	Carb	Fib	Tot. Fat	Sat. Fat	Chol	Sodium
110	6g	7g	1g	7g	4g	21mg	40mg

Apple Fritters

These are delicious served plain or topped with Blackberry Sauce, page 214.

1-1/4 cups all-purpose flour
2 tablespoons sugar
1 teaspoon baking powder
1 cup milk
1 tablespoon extra-light olive oil
2 egg whites
3 apples, peeled, cored, sliced
3 to 4 tablespoons extra-light olive oil for frying
Powdered sugar, if desired

Combine flour, sugar, baking powder, milk, and oil in a medium bowl, blender, or food processor; mix until blended. Beat egg whites and fold into batter. Stir apple slices into batter.

In a large skillet, heat oil over medium-high heat. For each fritter, carefully spoon about 2 tablespoons mixture into oil. When edges begin to brown, turn and cook other side. Place on absorbent paper or paper towels to drain excess oil. Cover and keep warm. Continue cooking remaining batter, adding more oil if necessary. Sprinkle with sifted powdered sugar, if desired. Makes about 20 fritters.

Each fritter contains:

Cal	Prot	Carb	Fib	Tot. Fat	Sat. Fat	Chol	Sodium
78	2g	11g	1g	3g	1g	2mg	23mg

Blackberry Sauce

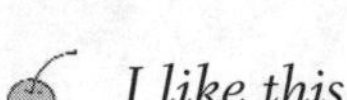

I like this sauce best with Apple Fritters, but it's also wonderful over sliced peaches or a scoop of ice cream.

2 cups fresh blackberries or 1 (12-oz.) package thawed, frozen, unsweetened blackberries
1/2 cup sugar
1/4 cup Frangelico (hazelnut liqueur) or orange juice
1/4 cup roasted hazelnuts, chopped

Crush blackberries or pulse in a food processor. Press through a strainer to remove seeds. Discard seeds and place pulp in a small saucepan; stir in sugar. Cook over low heat, stirring, until sugar is dissolved. Remove from heat and stir in Frangelico liqueur and hazelnuts. Serve warm or cold. Makes 2-1/2 cups.

Each tablespoon contains:

Cal	Prot	Carb	Fib	Tot. Fat	Sat. Fat	Chol	Sodium
20	0g	4g	0g	0g	0g	0mg	0mg

DRIED FRUIT COMPOTE

Serve this easy dessert during the winter months when fresh fruit is not available.

1 cup dried apricots
1 cup dried pears
1/4 cup raisins
1 cup apple juice
1 cup orange juice or water
1 tablespoon grated orange peel
1/2 cup dates, halved
1/2 cup plain fat-free yogurt
1 teaspoon grated nutmeg

Combine apricots, pears, raisins, apple juice, and orange juice or water in a saucepan. Gently simmer dried fruits until they are plumped and still hold their shape, 15 to 20 minutes. Add dates and cook 5 minutes. Serve warm fruit and juice in dessert bowls. Top with a dollop of yogurt and a sprinkle of nutmeg. Makes 6 servings.

Each serving contains:

Cal	Prot	Carb	Fib	Tot. Fat	Sat. Fat	Chol	Sodium
201	3g	50g	5g	1g	1g	0mg	23mg

FRUIT MEDLEY WITH HONEY-YOGURT SAUCE

Fresh fruits abound throughout the Mediterranean countries and are consumed at the peak of ripeness.

2 oranges, peeled, sliced
2 fresh pears, peeled, cored, sliced
24 green grapes
1 apple, unpeeled, cored, sliced
1 banana, peeled, sliced
2 tablespoons fresh lemon juice
16 strawberries, for garnish
Honey-Yogurt Sauce:
    1/4 cup honey
    3/4 cup plain fat-free yogurt
    2 tablespoons orange juice
    1 tablespoon grated orange peel

In a large bowl, combine oranges, pears, grapes, apple, and banana. Drizzle lemon juice over fruit and gently stir to combine. Spoon into serving dishes.

To make sauce, combine all ingredients in a small bowl. Top fruit with sauce. Garnish with strawberries. Makes 4 servings.

Each serving contains:

Cal	Prot	Carb	Fib	Tot. Fat	Sat. Fat	Chol	Sodium
237	4g	56g	7g	2g	1g	6mg	24mg

Oranges and Raspberries with Mascarpone

If navel or blood oranges are available, use them in this dessert. You may substitute pomegranate seeds for raspberries.

3 oranges, peeled, sliced
1/2 cup mascarpone cheese
1/4 cup whole milk or light cream
1 tablespoon Limoncello (lemon liqueur, optional)
1 cup red raspberries
1/4 cup chopped walnuts

Arrange orange slices on 4 dessert plates. In a cup, stir mascarpone, milk or cream, and liqueur (if using) together. Spoon over oranges and top with raspberries and walnuts. Makes 4 servings.

Each serving contains:

Cal	Prot	Carb	Fib	Tot. Fat	Sat. Fat	Chol	Sodium
385	8g	22g	6g	32g	15g	75mg	40mg

Café au Lait Pudding

If you desire stronger coffee flavor, use espresso coffee.

4 tablespoons cornstarch
1/2 cup sugar
1 cup double-strength cold coffee
1 cup half-and-half
1 teaspoon vanilla extract
Whipped cream (optional)

In a saucepan, blend together cornstarch and sugar. Add coffee and stir until cornstarch is dissolved. Add half-and-half and blend together. Cook over medium heat, stirring constantly, until thickened, 5 to 7 minutes. Remove from heat and stir in vanilla extract. If desired, serve with a dollop of whipped cream, if using. Makes 4 servings.

Each serving contains:

Cal	Prot	Carb	Fib	Tot. Fat	Sat. Fat	Chol	Sodium
131	0g	33g	0g	0g	0g	0mg	2mg

Lemon Gelato

This frozen treat has an intense flavor. Serve alone or with cantaloupe and Hazelnut Biscotti, page 220. If you like, substitute orange juice concentrate for the lemonade.

1/2 cup frozen lemonade concentrate
1 cup water
1 teaspoon grated lemon peel
2 cups half-and-half
3/4 cup light corn syrup

In a bowl, stir all ingredients together. Taste for sweetness; if too tart, add a little more corn syrup. Pour mixture into an ice-cream freezer container. Freeze according to manufacturer's directions. Makes 4 servings.

Each serving contains:

Cal	Prot	Carb	Fib	Tot. Fat	Sat. Fat	Chol	Sodium
397	4g	70g	0g	14g	9g	45mg	127mg

Hazelnut Biscotti

For special occasions, frost one side with melted chocolate bits.

6 tablespoons unsalted butter, softened
3/4 cup sugar
2 eggs
2-1/4 cups all-purpose flour
1-1/2 teaspoons baking powder
1/4 teaspoon salt
1 tablespoon grated lemon peel
2 tablespoons Frangelico (hazelnut liqueur)
1/4 cup Zante currants
1/2 cup roasted hazelnuts, chopped
1/2 cup roasted almonds, chopped

Preheat oven to 325°F (165°C). Grease and flour a baking sheet. In a mixer bowl, cream butter and sugar. Add eggs, one at a time, and beat well. In a bowl, stir together flour, baking powder, and salt. With mixer running on low speed, slowly add flour mixture and remaining ingredients. Divide dough in half. With floured hands, shape each half into a loaf; place loaves 3 inches apart on prepared baking sheet. Pat loaves to 2-1/2 inches wide and about 12 inches long.

Bake 25 to 30 minutes. Remove and cool loaves about 5 minutes. With a serrated knife, cut diagonally into 1/2-inch-thick slices. Return slices to baking sheet and bake again for 10 minutes. Cool before storing in a container with a tight-fitting lid. Makes 24 slices.

Each serving contains:

Cal	Prot	Carb	Fib	Tot. Fat	Sat. Fat	Chol	Sodium
136	3g	18g	1g	6g	2g	26mg	45mg

Almond Cookies

Spain is known for its wonderful almonds. These tender cookies almost melt in your mouth. Almonds are a good source of calcium.

1 cup unsalted butter, softened
1 cup powdered sugar
1-1/4 cups ground almonds
2 cups all-purpose flour
1 tablespoon vanilla extract

Preheat oven to 325°F (165°C). In a mixer bowl, beat together butter and sugar until well blended. Slowly blend in remaining ingredients. With floured hands, shape into 1-inch balls and place on a 15 x 10-inch parchment-lined or an ungreased nonstick baking sheet. Bake 15 to 18 minutes; cookies will not brown but will become firmer. Makes about 48 cookies.

Each cookie contains:

Cal	Prot	Carb	Fib	Tot. Fat	Sat. Fat	Chol	Sodium
86	1g	7g	1g	6g	3g	10mg	1mg

Chestnut and Apricot Parfait

Indulge yourself and enjoy an ice cream specialty that can be assembled in minutes.

3/4 cup chestnut purée
1 tablespoon pure rum extract
1/4 cup sugar
3 tablespoons chocolate syrup
1(15-oz.) can apricot halves, drained, chopped
1 pint light, sugar-free vanilla ice cream

In a small bowl, beat together chestnut purée, rum extract, sugar, and chocolate syrup. When blended, spoon into a pastry bag.

Chill parfait glasses in a freezer about 30 minutes before assembling dessert. Make two alternating layers of vanilla ice cream with about 1 tablespoon piped chestnut mixture and apricots. Serve at once or cover with plastic wrap and return to freezer about 3 hours until firm. Makes 8 servings.

Each serving contains:

Cal	Prot	Carb	Fib	Tot. Fat	Sat. Fat	Chol	Sodium
125	2g	43g	2g	2g	1g	5mg	44mg

ORANGE-WALNUT SEMOLINA CAKE

Not too sweet, this cake is ideal to accompany hot chocolate or coffee. Serve plain or with fresh berries or fruit.

1/3 cup extra-light olive oil
3/4 cup sugar
2 eggs
1/2 cup semolina flour (see Note below)
3/4 cup all-purpose flour
1 tablespoon baking powder
1/4 teaspoon salt (optional)
6 tablespoons orange juice
1 tablespoon grated orange peel
1/4 cup chopped walnuts
2 egg whites, beaten, stiff but not dry
Powdered sugar (optional)

Preheat oven to 350°F (180°C). Butter and flour a 9-inch-square baking pan; set aside. In a mixer bowl, thoroughly beat together oil, sugar, and eggs; continue beating about 5 minutes. Combine semolina, all-purpose flour, baking powder, and salt, if using. With mixer running, add dry ingredients to mixture alternately with orange juice. Fold in orange peel, walnuts, and beaten egg whites.

Pour into prepared pan and smooth top. Bake 30 to 35 minutes, or until top springs back when lightly pressed. Cool in pan. Slice and serve plain or top with a sprinkling of sifted powdered sugar. Makes 12 servings.

Each serving contains:

Cal	Prot	Carb	Fib	Tot. Fat	Sat. Fat	Chol	Sodium
181	3g	25g	1g	8g	1g	0mg	77mg

Note: Semolina flour is coarsely ground durum (high-protein) wheat. It can be purchased in natural food stores and some supermarkets.

Hazelnut and Currant Cake Topped with Lemon-Frangelico Syrup

A delicious special-occasion dessert, this cake is also delicious as an afternoon snack.

1 egg
3/4 cup sugar
1/4 cup extra-light olive oil
1/2 cup ground roasted hazelnuts
1/2 cup whole-wheat flour
1-1/4 cups all-purpose flour
1 tablespoon baking powder
2 tablespoons orange juice
2 tablespoons Frangelico (hazelnut liqueur)
1/2 cup milk
2 egg whites, beaten, stiff but not dry
1/3 cup Zante currants
Syrup:
1 cup water
3/4 cup sugar
1 tablespoon fresh lemon juice
1 tablespoon Frangelico (hazelnut liqueur)

Preheat oven to 350°F (175°C). Butter and flour a 9-inch-round baking pan; set aside. In a mixer bowl, thoroughly blend egg, sugar, and oil. In a bowl, combine hazelnuts, whole-wheat flour, all-purpose flour, and baking powder. In a cup, combine orange juice, Frangelico, and milk.

With mixer running, add dry ingredients to mixture alternately with orange juice mixture. Fold in egg whites and currants. Pour into prepared pan. Bake 35 to 40 minutes, or until top springs back when pressed. Cool 5 minutes before removing from pan and place on a cake rack.

While cake bakes, make syrup: Combine water, sugar, and lemon juice in a small saucepan; bring to a boil. Continue boiling 10 minutes. Remove from heat and stir in Frangelico. Set aside to cool.

With a fork, pierce cake top all over and spoon cooled syrup over top. Makes 12 servings.

Each serving of cake with syrup contains:

Cal	Prot	Carb	Fib	Tot. Fat	Sat. Fat	Chol	Sodium
257	4g	45g	1g	6g	1g	0mg	78mg

Index

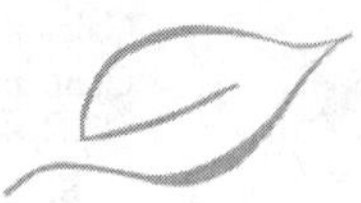

C

D

E

F

G

H–I

P

R

S

T

U–V

W

Y–Z